The Robotic Revolution in Hepatic Surgery

From Pioneering Scopes to Precision Healing

Ahmad Mahamid

Dedication

This book is dedicated to the memory of my father, whose belief in my path as an HPB surgeon I carry with me daily. It is for my dear mother, whose love has been a constant source of strength. And to my wife and children, my greatest support and inspiration.

It is also dedicated to the patients whose trust and courage inspire every medical advancement. Finally, I dedicate this to the pioneers of surgical robotics—the visionary engineers, developers, and intrepid surgeons whose pursuit of excellence has transformed the landscape of medicine and brought us to this era of precision healing.

Acknowledgment

Crafting "The Robotic Revolution in Hepatic Surgery" has been a journey deeply informed by the collective advancements and unwavering dedication of countless individuals across the globe. This book stands as a testament to the progress achieved in this complex and evolving field.

First and foremost, my deepest gratitude extends to the patients worldwide who have entrusted their care to innovative surgical approaches. Their courage and resilience are the ultimate inspiration behind every medical advancement.

I wish to acknowledge the pioneering engineers and developers whose groundbreaking work in robotics transformed theoretical concepts into tangible surgical platforms. Their vision and relentless pursuit of technological excellence have laid the foundation for the precision and capabilities we now see in the operating room.

My sincere appreciation goes out to the global community of hepatobiliary and robotic surgeons. Their tireless efforts in developing, refining, and teaching complex robotic techniques have been instrumental in pushing the boundaries of what's possible in liver surgery. The shared knowledge, published research, and collaborative spirit within this international surgical family are the bedrock upon which this book's content is built.

To the dedicated multidisciplinary teams – including anesthesiologists, intensivists, nurses, surgical assistants, and allied health professionals – who support every robotic liver procedure, your expertise and commitment to patient care are invaluable. The successful outcomes discussed in these pages are a direct reflection of your critical contributions in the operating room and throughout the patient's recovery journey.

I am also grateful to the medical researchers and librarians around the world whose diligent work in compiling, analyzing, and disseminating scientific literature provides the essential evidence base for surgical practice and innovation.

Finally, and most personally, I wish to thank my family and loved ones for their steadfast support, understanding, and encouragement. Their unwavering presence created the space and time necessary to bring this ambitious project to fruition.

This book is offered as a contribution to the ongoing global dialogue in robotic hepatic surgery, honoring the immense collective effort that continues to advance this life-saving specialty.

Table of Contents

Foreword

In the annals of surgical history, moments of profound transformation are rare, yet they redefine the very essence of patient care. We stand today at such a juncture, witnessing the breathtaking evolution of robotic technology that has reshaped, and continues to reshape the landscape of hepatic surgery. For decades, liver resection, a procedure fraught with complexity and demanding the utmost precision, has been the domain of skilled hands navigating through intricate anatomy, whether in open fields or via the narrow confines of laparoscopy. While these traditional approaches have served countless patients admirably, the inherent challenges—from managing blood loss and achieving oncological clearance to minimizing patient morbidity—have persistently driven surgeons to seek new frontiers.

This book, "The Robotic Revolution in Hepatic Surgery: From Pioneering Scopes to Precision Healing," serves as a vital chronicle of this extraordinary journey. It meticulously traces the trajectory of robotic platforms, from their nascent, experimental stages to their current embodiment as sophisticated instruments of unparalleled accuracy. We delve into the early visionaries who dared to dream of telemanipulation, the engineering marvels that brought these dreams to fruition, and the pioneering surgeons who first embraced these tools to navigate the delicate architecture of the liver. What began as a cautious exploration has blossomed into a robust and rapidly expanding field. Robotic liver surgery now routinely tackles complex resections, offering patients the benefits of minimally invasive approaches—reduced pain, shorter hospital stays, and faster recovery—without compromising oncological efficacy. This text not only celebrates these achievements but also critically examines the challenges overcome, the lessons learned, and the continued pursuit of excellence.

For surgical residents embarking on their careers, seasoned hepatobiliary surgeons seeking to integrate cutting-edge techniques, and anyone fascinated by the relentless march of medical innovation, this book offers an indispensable guide. It is a testament to human ingenuity and the collaborative spirit that drives medicine forward, promising a future where precision healing in hepatic surgery becomes the standard, not the exception.

Introduction: The Dawn of a New Era in Liver Surgery

The human liver, a metabolic powerhouse and the largest internal organ, presents unique and formidable challenges to the surgeon. Its intricate vascular and biliary anatomy, soft and highly vascularized parenchyma, and vital regenerative capacity demand unparalleled precision and a nuanced understanding during surgical intervention. For centuries, diseases affecting the liver, from primary and metastatic malignancies to benign conditions and trauma, have necessitated complex surgical resections. Historically, these procedures were characterized by extensive open incisions, significant blood loss, prolonged recovery periods, and substantial postoperative morbidity. Even with meticulous surgical technique, the sheer invasiveness of traditional open liver surgery carried inherent risks, including increased pain, higher rates of wound complications, and a prolonged return to normal activity, all of which underscored the imperative for less invasive yet equally effective approaches.

The latter half of the 20th century witnessed a transformative shift with the advent of minimally invasive surgery. Laparoscopy, initially embraced for simpler procedures like cholecystectomy, gradually expanded its reach to more complex abdominal operations, including early forays into hepatic resection. This represented a significant leap forward, offering patients the undeniable benefits of reduced pain, smaller scars, and quicker recovery compared to open approaches. However, despite its advantages, laparoscopic liver surgery inherently retains certain limitations, particularly when confronted with the liver's profound complexity. The rigid, linear instruments, the counter-intuitive fulcrum effect, the two-dimensional monoscopic vision (in early systems), and the complete absence of haptic feedback posed considerable technical hurdles. These limitations were particularly pronounced for intricate maneuvers like meticulous parenchymal transection, precise vascular control, and complex intracorporeal suturing within the delicate and highly vascular hepatic milieu. Consequently, major or centrally located laparoscopic liver resections, while feasible for a select cadre of expert hands, remained a formidable undertaking, often associated with a steep learning curve and a higher threshold for widespread adoption. The unmet needs in traditional liver surgery, even with the advent of laparoscopy, continued to drive the search for further technological advancements that could truly elevate precision and patient safety.

It was against this backdrop of persistent surgical challenges and the relentless pursuit of superior patient outcomes that robotic surgery emerged, signaling a profound paradigm shift in minimally invasive techniques. Initially conceived for telemanipulation in hazardous environments, such as remote military operations or space exploration, the application of robotics to the operating theatre began to gather significant momentum in the late 1990s. The promise was alluring and transformative: enhanced dexterity through wristed instruments that mimic the human hand's seven degrees of freedom, providing unparalleled articulation within confined spaces; immersive three-dimensional high-definition visualization that offers depth perception superior to traditional laparoscopy; and improved ergonomic comfort for the surgeon, potentially mitigating the physical strain and fatigue associated with prolonged, complex procedures. This new technological platform, spearheaded by systems like the da Vinci Surgical System, offered a level of control and precision previously unattainable in minimally invasive settings. For the liver, a highly vascular and parenchymatous organ where every millimeter of dissection and every ligated vessel carries critical implications, these technological advantages held particular significance. The ability to achieve fine dissection, precise vessel control, and meticulous parenchymal transection with greater stability, tremor filtration, and articulation offered a compelling new avenue for minimally invasive hepatic resection. The enhanced features directly addressed the inherent limitations of conventional laparoscopy, particularly for procedures situated deep within the abdominal cavity, in challenging posterior-superior segments, or those requiring complex suturing, reconstruction, and meticulous lymphadenectomy. The liver, with its demanding anatomical and physiological characteristics, thus became a prime candidate for robotic innovation, promising to expand the indications for minimally invasive surgery to a wider range of patients and pathologies, even the most complex.

"The Robotic Revolution in Hepatic Surgery: From Pioneering Scopes to Precision Healing" undertakes a comprehensive and deeply scientific journey through this remarkable evolution. This book aims to provide an evidence-based exploration, meticulously tracing the trajectory from the fundamental conceptualization of surgical robotics and its initial general surgical applications to its current cutting-edge and highly specialized use in hepatic surgery. We will delve into the foundational technologies that made this revolution possible, chronicle the pioneering surgical efforts that first dared to apply robotics to the liver, and systematically examine the expansion of indications for robotic liver resections, from basic resections to complex major hepatectomies and resections for demanding malignancies. Furthermore, this text will meticulously analyze the accumulated outcomes, including safety, efficacy, and oncological results, and critically project the exciting future directions that promise even greater precision, integration of artificial intelligence, and enhanced patient benefits. Serving as a definitive resource for trainees and seasoned practitioners alike, this book illuminates how robotics has not merely augmented, but profoundly revolutionized, the practice of liver surgery, ushering in an era of unprecedented precision and improved healing and setting the stage for the next wave of innovation in this vital specialty.

Part I: Foundations and Early Beginnings of Robotic Surgery

Chapter 1: The Genesis of Surgical Robotics

The continuous quest for enhanced precision, coupled with an unwavering drive for reduced invasiveness, has profoundly shaped the historical evolution of surgical practice. A truly transformative revolution in surgical technique gained significant and undeniable momentum during the latter half of the 20th century, specifically with the pioneering integration of advanced robotic systems into the operating theatre (1,2). This pivotal chapter delves into the foundational concepts that underpinned this profound revolution in surgery. It diligently traces the intricate trajectory of the early technological advancements that made such a shift possible. Furthermore, it chronicles the very initial introduction of these sophisticated robotic platforms into the broader domain of general surgical applications. This early and foundational adoption across various surgical disciplines established crucial precedents and technological pathways that would later prove indispensable for the profound and transformative impact of robotics on complex Hepato-Pancreato-Biliary (HPB) surgery. The overarching journey, spanning from rudimentary telemanipulation systems to the highly advanced and intelligent surgical robots of today, marks nothing less than a significant paradigm shift within the surgical field, consistently offering unprecedented levels of control and precision in the operating theatre (3).

1.1 Early Concepts and Visionaries: From Telemanipulation to Surgical Robots

The deepest conceptual roots of surgical robotics are firmly established and inextricably linked to the realm of telemanipulation. This innovative technological concept is fundamentally defined by its inherent ability to enable the precise control of a machine from a significant geographical or physical distance. The underlying principle of telemanipulation was not initially conceived for medical applications, but rather for its initial exploration and development in critical scenarios within hazardous environments. Such demanding and often dangerous settings, including specialized areas like nuclear facilities, presented inherent and undeniable risks where direct human presence was either completely impractical, exceedingly dangerous, or outright unsafe (2).

The fundamental idea that drove these seminal early explorations was the compelling and urgent need to extend the inherent dexterity and overall operational capability of human operators through the strategic and ingenious utilization of sophisticated mechanical interfaces. This groundbreaking approach was designed to allow highly complex and intricate tasks to be performed both safely and effectively from a remote location. These early prototypes, which were often generically referred to as "master-slave" systems, functioned on a reciprocal and highly intuitive control mechanism. In such a system, a human operator would meticulously control a "master" console, which would then precisely articulate the movements of a distant "slave" robotic arm (2,4). This fundamental operational principle effectively established the core concept of dexterity transfer and the creation of a tangible remote presence for the operator, qualities that would later define robotic surgery. This innovative paradigm allowed for human skill to be projected and applied into otherwise inaccessible or physically demanding anatomical spaces (2,4).

Development of surgical support robots began in the 1980s, initially conceived as navigation and auxiliary devices specifically designed to assist in endoscopic surgery (4). Visionary engineers, working in close collaboration with pioneering medical professionals, rapidly recognized the profound and transformative potential inherent in such burgeoning robotic technology (1). Their overarching aim was to significantly augment the physical capabilities of surgeons. This augmentation was critical for enhancing precision, particularly within confined anatomical spaces, and for effectively overcoming inherent human physiological limitations in surgery, such as involuntary physiological tremor and the onset of fatigue during prolonged procedures. The ultimate objective of integrating these advanced machines was not to replace the surgeon's indispensable cognitive decision-making processes, but rather to fundamentally transform the machines themselves into highly sophisticated extensions of the surgeon's own hands, thereby augmenting their physical capabilities to an unprecedented degree (1). Robotic surgery, in essence, emerged as a direct evolution of minimally invasive surgery, seamlessly combining elements of medical science, advanced robotics, and precision engineering (5).

The pivotal transition from these abstract theoretical concepts to practical medical applications witnessed the emergence of several early robotic prototypes. For instance, the PUMA 560 robot was notably utilized for a brain biopsy procedure conducted in 1985 (5). While initial surgical robot applications were diverse, these successful pioneering efforts laid the indispensable groundwork for the broader and more widespread adoption of robotic technology in later surgical contexts.

1.2 The Evolution of Robotic Systems: Da Vinci and Beyond

The true proliferation and widespread commercialization of surgical robotics commenced definitively with the strategic introduction of highly integrated platforms specifically designed for broad clinical utility and widespread adoption (6). Among these pioneering and commercially available systems, the da Vinci Surgical System rapidly emerged as a singularly dominant force within the rapidly expanding global robotic surgery market (4,7,8). This quintessential master-slave surgical support robot was meticulously developed during the latter half of the 1990s (4).

It achieved its initial pivotal United States Food and Drug Administration (FDA) approval for general laparoscopic surgical procedures in July 2000(6,9). This specific regulatory milestone held immense and lasting significance, as it formally signaled the widespread acceptance and irreversible integration of robot-assisted surgery into mainstream clinical practice across the United States. Following this critical U.S. regulatory acceptance, the da Vinci system also received broader international regulatory approval, including a notable endorsement in Japan in 2009 (4).

The da Vinci system was specifically engineered to directly address and overcome many of the inherent limitations that characterized conventional laparoscopic surgery. A cornerstone of its design was the provision of a high-resolution, three-dimensional (3D) magnified field of view. This advanced visualization capability dramatically improved depth perception, offering a distinct advantage when compared to the traditional 2D monoscopic vision typically available in early laparoscopic systems. Crucially, the da Vinci system incorporated sophisticated articulated "endo-wrist" instruments. These instruments were designed to mimic the natural dexterity and expansive seven degrees of freedom characteristic of the human hand and wrist. This revolutionary design allowed for the execution of exceptionally complex maneuvers, such as fine dissection and highly precise suturing, even within the most confined anatomical spaces. Furthermore, the system meticulously incorporated advanced tremor-filtering technology and highly effective motion scaling functions. These functionalities translated larger, often less precise, hand movements from the surgeon's console into smaller, more stable, and exquisitely precise instrument movements within the patient's body, thereby significantly enhancing overall surgical precision. These collective features also provided substantial ergonomic improvements for the operating surgeon, offering the potential to mitigate physical strain and reduce fatigue during prolonged and intricate surgical procedures (1,6,10)(4).

The da Vinci platform has undergone continuous and iterative development since its inception, with the da Vinci Xi representing its advanced fourth generation (4). This ongoing evolution in robotic system design has consistently aimed to promote superior surgical performance and effectively reduce the physical and mental workload experienced by surgeons (7). As experience with robotic technology matured and its diverse applications to advanced laparoscopic procedures became more thoroughly understood, a steadily increasing number of surgical procedures began to be performed with robotic assistance (6).

Initially, robotic-assisted laparoscopic cholecystectomy was widely recognized and deemed safe for routine practice. Subsequently, robotics demonstrated its safety and efficacy in a range of foregut procedures, including Nissen fundoplication, Heller myotomy, gastric banding procedures, and Roux-en-Y gastric bypass. These techniques honed in these procedures were then successfully extrapolated to other solid-organ operations, such as splenectomy, adrenalectomy, and pancreatic surgery, as well as complex robotic-assisted laparoscopic colectomy (6). Robotic surgery has indeed revolutionized the field of urology, enabling surgeons to perform complex procedures with greater precision and accuracy (11). Robotic-assisted hysterectomy for benign conditions was associated with a shorter hospital stay, less blood loss, and fewer complications compared to the open approach, with the main benefit of a shorter hospital stay when compared to laparoscopic and vaginal approaches (12,13). In the context of inguinal hernia repair, robotic approaches demonstrated similar safety parameters and postoperative outcomes to laparoscopic procedures (14). Robotic surgery also showed promise in complex cases of endometriosis, particularly those requiring significant resection, such as deep infiltrating endometriosis, due to benefits in managing lesion heterogeneity, predicting surgical complexity, and prolonged operative times in intricate scenarios (15,16). Furthermore, robot-assisted reconstruction techniques for ureteral strictures demonstrated superior functional outcomes, fewer postoperative complications, and faster recovery compared to open surgery(17). This broad and rapid expansion across numerous general surgical specialties underscored the versatility and technical advantages of the robotic platform.

Beyond the singular dominance of the da Vinci system, the rapid and dynamic growth in the field of surgical robotics has fostered the development and subsequent introduction of numerous other multi-visceral robotic systems. This proliferation signifies an important evolutionary phase in minimally invasive surgery, characterized by increasing competition and a robust drive towards further innovation within the robotic surgery landscape (18). Notably, other early robotic systems that received FDA approval and contributed to the expanding landscape included the ZEUS Robotic Surgical

System(6). AESOP, another robotic system by Computer Motion, addressed specific intraoperative needs by functioning as a robotic camera holder, thereby enhancing visualization stability (6). The introduction of the ZEUS robotic surgical system further advanced the capability to remotely operate laparoscopic instruments (6). More contemporary examples of these novel multi-port robotic surgical systems that have been introduced into clinical practice include Micro Hand S, Senhance, Revo-i MSR-5000, KangDuo, Versius, and Hugo™ RAS (19). This diversification reflects a robust and continuously evolving market actively seeking to provide alternative platforms and to consistently push the boundaries of robotic surgical capabilities even further.

1.3 Key Technological Advancements Paving the Way for Minimally Invasive Surgery

The successful and widespread integration of robotics into surgical practice was not an isolated technological event, but rather a direct and inevitable consequence of, and was further powerfully propelled by, a series of foundational technological advancements that broadly defined minimally invasive surgery (MIS) (6). Laparoscopy, having achieved significant expansion and widespread adoption in minimally invasive techniques over approximately 16 years prior to the more recent robust robotic developments, fundamentally introduced the core concept of performing complex surgical procedures through small, keyhole incisions (6)(20). This approach offered a suite of compelling patient benefits, including notably reduced postoperative pain, a quicker return to oral intake, significantly shorter hospitalizations, and impressively improved cosmetic results.

However, the initial laparoscopic systems, including those that were initially applied for highly complex procedures such as liver resection, were inherently limited by certain persistent technical constraints. These limitations frequently encompassed the use of rigid, linear instruments that lacked the crucial articulation capabilities of the human wrist, leading to constrained maneuverability. Furthermore, early systems provided only a two-dimensional (2D) visual field, which significantly compromised the surgeon's depth perception, a critical element for precise dissection. The stability of the camera platform could also be an issue. Beyond these, the complete absence of haptic (tactile) feedback posed considerable and often formidable technical hurdles for executing highly intricate maneuvers, such as meticulous parenchymal transection, precise vascular control, and delicate intracorporeal suturing within sensitive and highly vascular environments like the hepatic milieu (10)(21).

Robotic surgical systems emerged as a direct and innovative technological response specifically designed to precisely address and effectively overcome these aforementioned limitations of conventional laparoscopy. Robot-assisted laparoscopy specifically provided substantial and measurable improvements in overall surgical handling capabilities. The distinct advantages inherently offered by this advanced technique included significantly improved dexterity, which directly translated into a measurable increase in surgical precision. Moreover, the robotic platform inherently provides the effective elimination of physiological tremor, thereby mitigating a common human limitation, and profoundly reduces surgeon fatigue, both of which are crucial factors during long and demanding operations. These enhanced capabilities were instrumental in facilitating the performance of more extended and technically challenging resections, including those of the liver (6,22).

Key technological advancements that underpinned this transformative shift encompassed highly enhanced instrumentation, such as articulated instruments (often referred to as "endo-wrists") that could faithfully mimic the natural range of motion and articulation of the human hand and wrist. The development of multi-degree-of-freedom (Multi-DOF) wrist mechanisms further demonstrated ongoing efforts in the field to combine unparalleled precision with significantly improved surgical accessibility (23). Improved visualization represented another critical and parallel area of advancement, prominently featuring 3D high-definition (HD) vision systems that restored and provided essential depth perception to the surgical field (10). This significant advantage in visualization even led to a broader professional consensus recommending the routine use of 3D vision in general laparoscopy as a robust means to potentially reduce overall operative time (24). Furthermore, the critical incorporation of advanced imaging modalities, such as indocyanine green (ICG) fluorescence imaging, provided a crucial and highly valuable intraoperative advantage. ICG fluorescence is particularly valuable for the precise and real-time recognition of complex vascular and biliary anatomy during surgery, enhancing safety and accuracy (25). These collective and synergistic technological leaps directly and effectively addressed the numerous technical hurdles inherent in traditional laparoscopic approaches, thereby significantly extending the viable and safe options for minimally invasive surgery to a broader spectrum of complex general surgical procedures, particularly those previously deemed too challenging and requiring intricate movements or access to anatomically difficult areas (26).

1.4 The Role of the US Military and NASA in Early Robotic Development

The foundational genesis and subsequent early developmental trajectory of surgical robotics are deeply and intrinsically interconnected with strategic national interests in remote operation and the advancement of sophisticated technological capabilities. The conceptual roots of telemanipulation, fundamentally defined as a technology that enables the precise control of a machine from a significant geographical or physical distance, were initially explored and cultivated for critical applications in hazardous environments. These demanding and often life-threatening environments frequently encompassed scenarios directly relevant to military operations or ambitious space exploration endeavors. In such contexts, direct human presence was either completely impractical, exceedingly dangerous, or, in many cases, outright unsafe (2).

The fundamental drive and compelling impetus behind these early explorations was the urgent and compelling need to extend the inherent dexterity and overall operational capability of human operators through the strategic and ingenious implementation of sophisticated mechanical interfaces. This pioneering approach was specifically designed to facilitate the safe, effective, and precise performance of highly complex and intricate tasks from a remote and protected location.

The early development was notably driven by the compelling goal of enabling surgeons to operate a robot from a console, particularly in the context of facilitating remote surgery on the battlefield. This inherent pursuit of advanced remote control and enhanced precision in challenging and often life-threatening scenarios directly influenced the foundational design and subsequent developmental pathways of early surgical robots (4).

The capabilities refined through these early teleoperation concepts, such as dexterity transfer and remote presence, were precisely what would later be adapted and optimized for the controlled environment of the operating theatre, demonstrating a clear lineage from defense and space-related technological innovation to civilian medical application. For instance, the very concept of controlling a surgical instrument remotely from a console, a hallmark of modern robotic surgery, directly parallels the needs identified for telemanipulation in hazardous or distant environments. The drive to perform complex tasks with precision, mitigate human physiological limitations (like tremor, especially over long distances), and enhance capabilities in constrained settings, all principles championed by military and space research, found fertile ground in the surgical field. This foundational impetus contributed significantly to the development of early surgical robots and subsequently, their specialized application in complex procedures such as those in HPB surgery. The growth of robot-assisted surgery in the liver has occurred in a stepwise approach, which is very different from the frenzy seen with the introduction of laparoscopic cholecystectomy. This stepwise approach allowed the identification of areas for improvement, many of which are at the nexus of engineering and medicine. Further improvements in robot-assisted surgery depend on the combined efforts of engineers and surgeons (27).

1.5 Ethical and Regulatory Considerations in the Adoption of New Surgical Technologies

The rapid and transformative introduction of robotic technology into surgical practice brought forth a complex and multifaceted array of ethical and regulatory considerations. As with any significant medical innovation, its widespread adoption necessitated a careful examination of its impact on patient care, surgical training, and healthcare economics (10).

Key concerns that prominently emerged revolved around ensuring the paramount aspect of patient safety. While the theoretical advantages of robotics in precision and control were compelling, robust evidence of improved safety over established methods was crucial for responsible integration. Additionally, significant attention was directed towards effectively managing the steep learning curve inherently associated with surgeons acquiring and mastering proficiency in these novel and complex robotic techniques (7). The need to ensure that surgeons could achieve competence without compromising patient outcomes was a central ethical challenge. Addressing the substantial financial costs involved in both acquiring and subsequently maintaining these advanced robotic systems also constituted a primary and pervasive concern (28). Furthermore, considerable controversy persisted within the broader medical community regarding the concrete economic benefits and the demonstrable real advantages for the patient when directly compared to existing conventional or established "gold standard" surgical approaches (8).

Regulatory bodies played a uniquely pivotal role in the comprehensive vetting and subsequent oversight of these nascent and rapidly evolving technologies. A landmark event in this crucial regulatory landscape was the United States Food and Drug Administration (FDA) approval of the da Vinci robotic surgical system in July 2000 (6). This specific approval further defined the capability of a robotic-assist device to effectively address and overcome some of the persistent limitations previously identified in conventional laparoscopy. This FDA authorization was a critical milestone, unequivocally signifying regulatory confidence in the system's fundamental safety and its demonstrable efficacy for a broad spectrum of general laparoscopic procedures (9).

However, challenges persisted throughout the early phases of widespread adoption. The comparability of currently available retrospective case studies for complex procedures, such as robotic liver resections, was notably difficult, often due to variations in methodologies and limited sample sizes (29). This highlighted a pressing and urgent need for larger, well-designed prospective studies and, crucially, randomized trials to comprehensively and definitively analyze the true value and long-term impact of robotic surgery (30). Despite the steadily increasing utilization of robotic surgery across a wide and diverse range of surgical procedures, concrete evidence specifically supporting consistently improved clinical outcomes after robotic surgery remained notably limited during its early stages of development and adoption. Consequently, a clear demand arose for more rigorous and methodologically sound research, explicitly focused on demonstrating tangible, patient-important benefits. Such evidence was deemed absolutely necessary before any further widespread expansion of robotic surgery could be responsibly pursued on a larger scale (30).

The inherent high cost associated with the use of the robotic system, primarily driven by the substantial purchase price of the unit, the ongoing maintenance expenses, and the high cost of disposable instruments, coupled with often longer operative times in the initial phases, remained a significant financial barrier that notably limited its widespread adoption (28). Moreover, the robotic platform often required added operating time associated with docking and instrument exchange. Nevertheless, for highly complex procedures such as robotic liver resections, the financial burden is observed to be relatively lower in high-volume centers. This lower cost can be partially offset by potential benefits such as more rapid patient recovery and a shorter hospital stay for robotic hepatectomy. Furthermore, this financial burden is generally expected to decrease in the near future as an increasing number of new surgical systems enter the market, fostering greater competition and potentially driving down overall costs (31)(8).

These ongoing ethical discussions, coupled with the continuous refinement of regulatory frameworks and surgeon training protocols, remain essential for the responsible and effective integration and sustained growth of robotic surgery within the evolving landscape of modern surgical practice. Concerns unique to robotic surgery, including safety protocols, must be diligently put in place and reviewed at the beginning of every procedure to ensure safety, particularly in the event of an emergent conversion to open surgery (32). Despite promising results, still large, multicenter, randomized, and prospective studies are needed to analyze the exact value of robotic liver surgery in patients with malignant liver tumors (22). The implementation of standardized education and certification for future generations of surgeons considering robotic surgery is also crucial to ensure patient safety (33).

Chapter 2: Initial Forays into Robotic Abdominal Surgery

The evolution of robotic surgery into the operating theater gained significant momentum in the late 1990s, building upon the foundational concepts of telemanipulation and master-slave systems established in earlier decades (2,4). This new technological platform, spearheaded by systems like the da Vinci Surgical System, offered a level of control and precision previously unattainable in minimally invasive settings (3). The da Vinci Surgical System received crucial regulatory approval in the United States in July 2000 for general laparoscopic procedures (6,9). This pivotal approval marked a significant shift, signaling the formal acceptance of robot-assisted surgery into mainstream clinical practice across various abdominal disciplines.

The initial foray of robotics into the abdominal cavity involved a cautious yet progressive expansion of its applications, addressing known limitations of conventional laparoscopy and seeking to improve patient outcomes. This period was characterized by a meticulous exploration of the robotic platform's capabilities across a diverse range of general surgical procedures, thereby establishing feasibility, accumulating initial experience, and confronting the inherent challenges of integrating advanced technology into complex human interventions. The lessons learned during these foundational years, particularly concerning learning curves, early clinical outcomes, technical limitations, and the economic implications, would prove indispensable in paving the way for the later, more specialized applications of robotics in intricate fields such as hepatobiliary (HPB) surgery. This chapter delves into these crucial early experiences, providing a comprehensive understanding of the initial trajectory of robotic abdominal surgery.

2.1 Early Applications and Expanding Scope in General Robotic Surgery

Following its foundational FDA approval, early applications of robotic surgery in general abdominal procedures primarily focused on relatively simpler operations, thereby establishing feasibility and accumulating initial experience. Robotic-assisted laparoscopic cholecystectomy, for instance, was among the first procedures widely recognized and deemed safe for routine practice using the robotic platform (6,34). Its adoption facilitated enhanced control, making it an early success story in minimally invasive surgery.

The scope of robotic application rapidly expanded beyond simple cholecystectomies to include a range of foregut procedures, such as Nissen fundoplication, Heller myotomy, gastric banding procedures, and Roux-en-Y gastric bypass (6,35). These early successes demonstrated the robotic system's inherent ability to safely execute established laparoscopic procedures while consistently offering enhanced control and precision in confined spaces. As experience with robotic technology matured and its diverse applications to advanced laparoscopic procedures became more thoroughly understood, a steadily increasing number of surgical procedures began to be performed with robotic assistance (6).

The techniques honed in these initial operations were successfully extrapolated to other solid-organ procedures, including splenectomy, adrenalectomy, and pancreatic surgery, as well as complex robotic-assisted laparoscopic colectomy. For example, robotic adrenalectomy consistently demonstrated feasibility and safety, achieving outcomes comparable to laparoscopic adrenalectomy in high-volume centers, driven by its greater precision and better ergonomics (10,36). Robotic appendicectomy was also found to be safe and feasible, characterized by minimal blood loss and acceptable operative time and hospital stay, highlighting its versatility in both elective and emergency settings (37).

The transformative impact of robotics extended significantly to colorectal surgery, where robotic procedures have been increasingly adopted, showing benefits such as reduced postoperative discomfort, shorter hospital stays, and accelerated recovery compared to open surgery (38,39). Robotic right hemicolectomy has been associated with a higher yield of harvested lymph nodes, a lower conversion rate to open surgery, a shorter time to flatus, and a shorter length of hospital stay (40). For gastric cancer, robotic gastrectomy has been increasingly employed to overcome some limitations of conventional laparoscopic gastrectomy, achieving better short-term surgical outcomes and a higher rate of retrieved lymph nodes (41,42). In Eastern countries, robotic gastrectomy is routinely employed for early-stage gastric cancer, indicating growing confidence in its safety and oncological adequacy (43).

Beyond the gastrointestinal tract, robotic surgery revolutionized the field of urology, enabling surgeons to perform complex procedures with greater precision and accuracy. Robotic-assisted radical prostatectomy, for instance, has been consistently linked to less estimated blood loss and shorter hospital stays, showcasing the advantages of minimally invasive techniques for complex resections (44). Robotic-assisted hysterectomy for benign conditions was associated with a shorter hospital stay, less blood loss, and fewer complications compared to the open approach, with the main benefit of a shorter hospital stay when compared to laparoscopic and vaginal approaches (12,13). In the context of inguinal hernia repair, robotic approaches demonstrated similar safety parameters and postoperative outcomes to laparoscopic procedures (14). Robotic surgery also showed promise in complex cases of endometriosis, particularly those requiring significant resection, such as deep infiltrating endometriosis, due to benefits in managing lesion heterogeneity, predicting surgical complexity, and handling prolonged operative times in intricate scenarios (15,16). Furthermore, robot-assisted reconstruction techniques for ureteral strictures demonstrated superior functional outcomes, fewer postoperative complications, and faster recovery compared to open surgery (17). This broad and rapid expansion across numerous general surgical specialties underscored the versatility and technical advantages of the robotic platform, laying crucial groundwork for its eventual and profound impact on hepatobiliary surgery.

2.2 Learning Curves and Skill Acquisition in Robotic Surgery

The successful and widespread implementation of robotic surgery programs across various institutions necessitated a comprehensive, multidisciplinary team approach, demanding significant commitment and investment from clinical faculty, operating room staff, and hospital administrators. This institutional commitment is foundational for creating an environment conducive to learning and safe practice, particularly given the recognized learning curve inherent in adopting new complex technologies. A period of dedicated practice and training is consistently required for surgeons to achieve proficiency with robotic systems (45–47).

To facilitate this demanding process, robotic surgical training requires systematization for young surgeons, aiming to standardize it and enable adaptation to a wider range of surgical applications (45). Structured training pathways have been developed to guide surgeons through the skill acquisition process. The European Hernia

Society, for example, describes a training curriculum for robot-assisted abdominal wall surgery that is contingent upon the specific robot platform, the surgeon's prior experience in other abdominal procedures, and their existing expertise in abdominal wall repair techniques. This framework typically encompasses both preclinical phases, involving didactic learning and simulation, and subsequent clinical phases, with the latter specifically focusing on the practical introduction of the robotic platform into surgical practice under supervision (48). This phased approach is crucial for safely navigating the learning curve in complex robotic procedures.

Some studies have indicated that the learning curve for specific robotic procedures, such as robotic right colectomy, can be significantly faster when compared to laparoscopic approaches (49). This suggests that the ergonomic and technical advantages of robotics, such as enhanced dexterity and 3D vision, may indeed accelerate the acquisition of certain psychomotor skills. However, the overall complexity of various surgical procedures means that while the robotic platform may offer a shortened learning curve for surgeons when compared to laparoscopic approaches for extensive operations (31), a substantial training period is still universally required for the complex decision-making and critical maneuvers unique to each specialty.

Simulation and virtual reality (VR) play a crucial and increasingly prominent role in skill acquisition for robotic surgery. Many robotic surgery curricula extensively utilize commercial virtual reality simulators as a primary component of their training programs (50). These advanced simulators are instrumental in aiding surgeons to learn basic robotics skills and to practice procedural activities effectively in a safe and controlled environment, thereby promoting effective skill development without patient risk. Video-based educational tools in robotic surgery have also demonstrably shown a positive effect on educational outcomes, proving particularly valuable for skill development when used as a review tool (51). The refinement of perioperative care through optimized surgical techniques and structured complication management has also contributed to improving outcomes in minimally invasive surgery, including robotic procedures. Ensuring patient safety through standardized education and certification for the future generation of surgeons considering robotic surgery is a critical measure, as the use of robots in surgery continues to expand (33).

2.3 Challenges and Limitations of Early Robotic Systems

Despite the numerous advantages and the promising expansion of its applications, early robotic systems presented inherent limitations that posed significant challenges to their widespread adoption and optimal utilization. Understanding these early hurdles is crucial for appreciating the subsequent refinements that have propelled robotic surgery forward.

A prominent technical hurdle lay in the design of the instruments themselves; early robotic systems often featured rigid, linear instruments that lacked the crucial articulation capabilities of the human wrist, which severely limited maneuverability within confined anatomical spaces. Furthermore, the initial visual interface often provided only a two-dimensional (2D) monoscopic view, which significantly compromised the surgeon's depth perception, a critical element for precise dissection and tissue manipulation. The stability of the camera platform, while generally improved over early laparoscopy, could still be an issue in some instances. Perhaps one of the most notable limitations was the complete absence of haptic (tactile) feedback, posing considerable and often formidable technical hurdles for executing highly intricate maneuvers, such as meticulous parenchymal transection, precise vascular control, and delicate intracorporeal suturing within sensitive and highly vascular environments like the hepatic milieu (31).

Beyond these technical constraints, the cost associated with robotic surgery presented a significant and pervasive barrier to its widespread adoption (28). Robotic adrenalectomy, for example, could be up to 2.3 times more costly than laparoscopic adrenalectomy, primarily due to the substantial purchase price and ongoing maintenance of the robotic unit, the high cost of disposable instruments, and often longer operative times in the initial phases

(10). These economic imperatives necessitated a thorough cost-benefit analysis of early robotic procedures. Studies consistently showed that while robotic surgery could achieve similar clinical outcomes, it frequently incurred higher costs and longer operative times compared to conventional laparoscopic approaches (14,28,42,52). The robotic platform also often required added operating time associated with docking and instrument exchange (31). The high cost and limited availability remained significant drawbacks for even seemingly straightforward procedures like appendicectomy (37).

Challenges also extended to the operational dynamics within the operating room. Workflow and teamwork could be impacted in robot-assisted surgery due to the surgeon being physically positioned away from the patient's bedside at a console. Studies focused on flow disruptions and non-technical skills identified communication breakdowns, coordination issues, and challenges related to training and equipment/technology as frequent causes of disruptions during robotic procedures (53). Furthermore, early evidence supporting consistently improved clinical outcomes after robotic surgery was noted as limited (30), and controversies about economic benefits and actual patient advantages over existing gold standards persisted (8). Early retrospective case studies were often difficult to compare due to methodological variations and small datasets, leading to urgent calls for larger, prospective, and randomized trials to analyze the true value and long-term impact of robotic surgery (8,29). Specific controversies continue to exist regarding robotic liver resection, despite its increasing application in recent years (54).

2.4 Patient Selection, Initial Clinical Outcomes, and Early Evidence Limitations

The early phases of robotic surgical application were crucial for establishing feasibility and understanding the initial clinical outcomes across a wide variety of general surgery procedures. Patient selection played a pivotal role in these early endeavors, as surgeons sought to identify appropriate cases where the nascent robotic technology could offer benefits without undue risk.

Initial robotic surgical applications successfully established the feasibility of this new approach across a wide variety of general surgery procedures (6). For instance, robot-assisted adrenalectomy consistently demonstrated both feasibility and safety, achieving outcomes comparable to traditional laparoscopic adrenalectomy in specialized, high-volume centers (10,55). Similarly, robotic appendicectomy was considered a safe and feasible option in both elective and emergency settings, characterized by minimal blood loss and acceptable operative time and hospital stay (37). Robot-assisted reconstruction techniques for ureteral strictures showcased superior functional outcomes, fewer postoperative complications, and a notably faster recovery period when directly compared to open surgical approaches (17).

In the rapidly evolving field of colorectal surgery, the safety, efficacy, and learning curve for most robotic applications have been progressively established, contributing to a steady growth in robot utilization (56). Robotic proctectomy, for example, exhibited a decrease in complications and an increase in the number of harvested lymph nodes as surgeon experience accumulated (57). Early studies comparing robotic and laparoscopic approaches for various procedures often showed similar safety parameters and overall postoperative outcomes, with the robotic platform offering some advantages in specific areas (6,30,58). For gastric cancer surgery, robotic gastrectomy was associated with longer operating time but also less intraoperative blood loss and a lower rate of surgical complications when compared to laparoscopic gastrectomy (42). Robotic-assisted hysterectomy, when compared to open approaches, was associated with shorter hospital stays, less blood loss, and fewer complications (13). For inguinal hernia repair, robotic approaches demonstrated safety parameters and postoperative outcomes similar to laparoscopic procedures(14). Robotic cholecystectomy, another early and widespread application, was characterized by minimal blood loss and acceptable operative time and hospital stay (34).

However, despite these promising initial outcomes and the demonstrated feasibility across numerous specialties, the quality of some early studies was generally noted to be low. The findings were often limited by the small size of the datasets utilized, and meaningful comparisons between studies on the same topic were frequently restricted due to significant heterogeneity in algorithms and datasets. This highlights a crucial limitation in the early evidence base, emphasizing that while feasibility was established, definitive long-term advantages often required more robust data.

2.5 The Economic Imperative: Cost-Benefit Analysis of Early Robotic Procedures

The economic considerations surrounding early robotic surgical procedures represented a significant and often prohibitive factor limiting their widespread adoption across healthcare systems. While robotic surgery frequently offered compelling clinical advantages, these benefits invariably had to be carefully weighed against the substantially increased costs associated with implementing and maintaining this advanced technology.

For instance, a meta-analysis comparing robotic and laparoscopic inguinal hernia repair explicitly found that overall costs were consistently higher in the robotic group (14). Similarly, in the context of gastrectomy for gastric cancer, despite the robotic approach showing some advantages in perioperative outcomes and lymph node retrieval, its high cost remained a significant barrier to broader implementation (41,42). More specifically, robotic adrenalectomy could be up to 2.3 times more costly than its laparoscopic counterpart(10). Even for seemingly less complex procedures like appendicectomy, the high cost and limited availability of robotic systems remained recognized drawbacks (37). This increased cost was primarily attributed to the considerable purchase price and ongoing maintenance expenses of the robotic unit, the high cost of specialized disposable instruments, and often longer operative times in the initial phases of adoption.

In the realm of emergency general surgery, while perioperative outcomes for robotic surgery might be comparable to laparoscopic surgery in selected conditions, the associated costs were notably and significantly higher (28,59). This underscored a broader concern that the financial investment might outweigh the demonstrated clinical benefits in certain settings. Studies conducting formal cost-utility analyses of robotic-assisted surgery generally yielded mixed results, highlighting the complexity of quantifying the economic value. While some analyses indicated that robotic surgery could indeed be more cost-effective than traditional open surgery for specific procedures, such as prostatectomy, colectomy, and gastrectomy, the evidence remained inconsistent when directly comparing it to laparoscopic surgery (60,61). This inconsistency suggested that further and more rigorous work was urgently needed on cost-utility analyses to fully understand the comprehensive economic benefits across different surgical contexts.

The high cost of surgical procedures, combined with the expense of equipment, instruments, and maintenance, were consistently identified as an important aspect to consider for sustainable adoption. The substantial costs of robot acquisition and maintenance could be partially offset by potential benefits such as more rapid patient recovery and a shorter hospital stay for robotic hepatectomy (31). Nevertheless, balancing the clinical advantages with the formidable economic imperative continued to be a central challenge in the early widespread adoption of robotic surgical platforms in abdominal surgery. The ongoing debate emphasizes the need for larger, standardized studies to better evaluate the impact of robotic surgery on surgical outcomes and its role in the future, justifying higher costs through patient care benefits.

Part II: The Emergence of Robotic Liver Surgery

Chapter 3: The Pioneering Years: First Robotic Liver Resections

The application of robotic technology to liver surgery represented a significant and transformative leap in the ongoing evolution of minimally invasive techniques for this complex and delicate organ. While laparoscopic liver surgery had already begun to demonstrate its considerable advantages, particularly in terms of reduced patient morbidity and accelerated recovery, conventional laparoscopic approaches inherently retained certain limitations(20). These persistent technical constraints included rigid instruments, a two-dimensional (2D) visual field compromising depth perception, and a notable absence of haptic (tactile) feedback, posing considerable technical hurdles for meticulous parenchymal transection, precise vascular control, and delicate intracorporeal suturing within the sensitive hepatic milieu (21). It was against this backdrop of persistent surgical challenges that robotic surgery emerged, promising to elevate precision and patient safety, particularly for demanding liver operations (22,62).

The growth of robot-assisted surgery in the liver has unfolded as a deliberate stepwise approach, which is notably different from the rapid and widespread adoption (often described as a "frenzy") observed with the introduction of laparoscopic cholecystectomy. This controlled, stepwise growth allowed for the identification of critical areas for improvement, many of which reside at the intricate nexus of advanced engineering and precise medical practice. Further improvements in robot-assisted surgery, therefore, depend significantly on the combined efforts of both engineers and surgeons (27). This chapter will meticulously chronicle the pioneering efforts that first dared to apply robotic technology to the liver, systematically examining the initial indications, the unique technical challenges encountered, the learning curve associated with these novel procedures, and the early comparisons with established laparoscopic approaches.

3.1 Initial Case Reports and Proving the Concept

The application of robotic technology to liver surgery marked a significant advancement in the evolution of minimally invasive techniques for this complex organ. The very first hepatectomy performed using a robotic approach was formally reported in 2002 (9). This seminal event occurred a full decade after the initial laparoscopic hepatectomy, highlighting the sequential progression of minimally invasive techniques in the hepatic field(9). In these early years of robotic hepatic surgery, comprehensive series documenting outcomes were notably scarce, and a general lack of robust and relevant data in the existing literature presented a significant obstacle to the more widespread development and acceptance of robot-assisted laparoscopic hepatectomy (RALH).

Nevertheless, the fundamental concept of performing liver resections with robotic assistance began to steadily gain traction, primarily driven by the compelling technical advantages offered by these nascent new platforms. These platforms, originating from concepts of telemanipulation and designed to overcome limitations of conventional laparoscopy, provided enhanced dexterity, three-dimensional (3D) visualization, and tremor filtration (21,22,25).

Such capabilities were particularly attractive for the intricate nature of liver surgery.

Early reports from major robotic-assisted pancreatic surgery series, which often share technical complexities and demanding anatomical requirements with liver resections due to their close anatomical proximity and intricate vascular and biliary connections, showed encouraging preliminary results. Pancreatic surgery itself is considered a challenging application of minimally invasive surgery. These reports, although not directly liver-focused, indicated that robotic pancreatectomy could achieve morbidity and mortality rates comparable to those of traditional open surgery, and preliminary data on cancer survival rates also appeared similar to open series. Such encouraging preliminary data in complex Hepato-Pancreato-Biliary (HPB) procedures provided a conceptual foundation and impetus for expanding robotic application to the liver (63).

A pioneering systematic review specifically focusing on robot-assisted major hepatectomy (defined as the resection of three or more liver segments) analyzed a total of 68 robotic major hepatectomies, which included 38 right hepatectomies and 30 left hepatectomies (64). Notably, this cohort of pioneering major robotic liver resections reported no deaths. Conversion to open surgery occurred in 5.2% of right hepatectomies and 3.3% of left hepatectomies in these early series. The weighted average operative time was 418.6 minutes and intraoperative blood loss was 411.4 mL. Only a small percentage of patients (6.3%) required blood transfusions, and 17 developed postoperative complications (26.9%). Information on tumor type was available for 57 patients, revealing that 42 patients (73.6%) were diagnosed with malignant tumors, while 15 patients (26.3%) presented with benign disease. No port site metastasis, peritoneal carcinomatosis, or intrahepatic recurrence were reported, and only three patients had microscopic margin positivity. These early case reports and small series were instrumental in demonstrating the fundamental feasibility of performing complex major resections under robotic assistance, even as further experience was acknowledged as necessary before definitive conclusions could be drawn. The da Vinci Surgical System, having demonstrated surgical feasibility since its market introduction in 2000, began to show its potential in complex robotic liver resections. The collective evidence, even from these nascent stages, suggested that robot-assisted hepatobiliary surgery was steadily growing and offered a viable alternative to both open and conventional laparoscopic approaches for selected patients. The success in expanding robot-assisted procedures to general surgery, including initial widespread applications like laparoscopic cholecystectomy, further paved the way for its adoption in more complex solid-organ procedures like those in the liver (6).

3.2 Technical Challenges Unique to Hepatic Robotics: Transection and Hemostasis

Liver surgery is inherently one of the most technically demanding applications within abdominal surgery due to the organ's highly complex anatomy, characterized by an intensive and intricately variant vascular and biliary system. Achieving precise parenchymal transection and meticulous hemostasis is absolutely critical during liver resections, given the highly vascular nature of the hepatic parenchyma. Traditional conventional laparoscopic liver resection, while representing a significant advance in minimally invasive surgery, presented significant inherent limitations in executing these critical steps (21,22).

These limitations frequently encompassed a reduced freedom of instrument movement within the confined abdominal cavity, and a limited 2-dimensional (2D) view of the operative field, which profoundly compromised depth perception. Furthermore, the complete absence of haptic (tactile) feedback in early laparoscopic systems posed considerable and often formidable technical hurdles for executing highly intricate maneuvers, such as meticulous parenchymal transection, precise vascular control, and delicate intracorporeal suturing within the sensitive and highly vascular hepatic milieu (21).

Robotic surgical systems emerged with the explicit aim to address and overcome many of these technical constraints inherent in conventional laparoscopy, thereby offering potential solutions to these complex challenges in liver surgery. Robot-assisted laparoscopy was designed to improve surgical handling. The distinct advantages inherently offered by this advanced technique include significantly improved dexterity, which directly translated into increased surgical precision, and the effective elimination of physiological tremor and reduction of surgeon fatigue. These enhanced capabilities were instrumental in facilitating the performance of more extended and technically challenging liver resections (1,21,22).

The introduction of EndoWrist instruments and enhanced visualization specifically provided important advantages in terms of selective bleeding control, facilitating micro-suturing, and enabling more precise dissection (25). The robotic platform also offers a three-dimensional (3D) view of the surgical site, which further improves depth perception and precision (21). However, despite these advancements, the robotic platform initially remained limited by a paucity of dedicated parenchymal transection devices and a complete lack of haptic feedback. Moreover, the robotic approach often involved added operating time associated with docking and instrument exchange, a factor that could prolong overall procedure duration (31).

Despite these early limitations, the use of robotic surgery for hepatic procedures originated precisely because of its technical potential to overcome several major technical limitations known from conventional laparoscopy. It offered the possibility of performing more extended liver resections in a minimally invasive fashion. Studies consistently showed that using the robotic technique was associated with a decreased or at least equal amount of intraoperative blood loss compared to that of the conventional laparoscopic or open technique. The increasing application of robotic liver resection has shown benefits in some aspects owing to the technical advancement of the robotic surgical system, though controversies still exist (22,31,32,54).

The advanced capabilities, such as increased dexterity from endo-wristed instruments, improved 3D vision, and computer filtration of surgeon's movements, specifically addressed the complexity of performing delicate reconstructions involving biliary, pancreatic, and enteric anastomoses, thereby bringing minimally invasive hepato-pancreato-biliary surgery into a new era (63). The anatomical understanding, particularly related to structures like the extrahepatic Glissonean pedicle and Laennec's capsule, would contribute to standardizing surgical techniques for anatomical liver resection, including laparoscopic or robotic liver resection, and bring innovative changes for spreading safe and curable liver resection (65).

3.3 Early Indications: Benign Lesions and Peripheral Resections

In the pioneering years of robotic liver surgery, initial applications primarily focused on less complex procedures and the resection of benign conditions. This cautious approach aimed to firmly establish the platform's fundamental feasibility, safety, and reproducibility before venturing into more complex oncological or anatomical indications. The strategy mirrored the earlier adoption of laparoscopy for simpler abdominal procedures like cholecystectomy, which then gradually expanded to more intricate operations.

Minor hepatectomies, which typically involve the resection of fewer than three liver segments, such as left-lateral sectionectomy and wedge resections of anterior segments, were among the first procedures to be widely accepted as the standard of care for laparoscopic approaches, and subsequently became common early indications for robotic adoption. These procedures served as a crucial proving ground for the robotic system in the hepatic context, allowing surgeons to gain familiarity with the robotic interface, enhanced visualization, and improved dexterity in a less physiologically demanding setting (66).

Early systematic reviews of robot-assisted major hepatectomy, which included major resections of three or more liver segments, analyzed a cohort of 68 robotic major hepatectomies. In this early experience, information on tumor types was available for 57 patients, revealing that 42 patients (73.6%) were diagnosed with malignant tumors, while 15 patients (26.3%) presented with benign diseases. This demonstrates that even in the early phases of major resections, a significant portion of cases involved benign pathologies, contributing to the initial safety profile data. These early experiences were instrumental in establishing the safety profile of robotic major resections for non-malignant indications, particularly when dealing with large or deeply situated benign lesions(64). Robotic surgery is indeed being utilized to treat a variety of benign conditions, and studies indicate no deterioration in outcomes when compared to other approaches (27).

When evaluated against open surgery, robotic resection for benign liver diseases has been associated with several quantifiable advantages, including a statistically lower incidence of blood loss, a shorter length of hospital stay, and a reduced overall complication rate (67). Although studies suggest that peri- and postoperative outcomes for robotic surgery are generally similar to those observed with laparoscopic surgery in this context, robotic platforms offer distinct advantages in overcoming specific technical limitations inherent in conventional laparoscopy. These limitations include constraints imposed by rigid instruments and a two-dimensional (2D) visual field, both of which are particularly restrictive when dealing with large or centrally located benign tumors. The enhanced visualization provided by robotic platforms, particularly three-dimensional (3D) high-definition (HD) vision, is crucial for accurately delineating complex benign lesions from healthy liver parenchyma and for meticulous dissection around critical vascular and biliary structure. This improved depth perception and magnification aid significantly in navigating the intricate vascular architecture often encountered with larger or highly vascular benign tumors, such as hemangiomas or large adenomas (21,25,67).

Robotic resection of the caudate lobe, a segment of the liver that is anatomically deeply located and maintains complex relationships with major vessels, is considered a highly challenging surgical procedure. However, robotic approaches have consistently demonstrated feasibility and safety for tumors situated in this difficult-to-access segment, including benign lesions, yielding promising postoperative outcomes (68). The ability of robotic systems to provide enhanced precision and maneuverability in such confined and critical anatomical spaces is a direct advantage. Similarly, robotic resections for lesions in the posterior-superior segments of the liver, which are notoriously difficult to access and manipulate effectively with conventional laparoscopic tools due to anatomical constraints, have proven feasible and safe (22). A meta-analysis comparing robotic versus laparoscopic liver resection for these challenging posterosuperior segments revealed that robotic liver resection was associated with less estimated blood loss, fewer blood transfusions, and shorter operative time, with comparable morbidity and mortality rates to laparoscopic approaches (69). This highlights the specific benefits of robotics for these anatomically demanding locations, which can frequently harbor benign lesions requiring resection.

Beyond the liver parenchyma itself, robotic surgery has also proven adept in managing complex benign pathologies within the broader HPB system, which often involve delicate dissection and reconstruction. Robotic-assisted cholecystectomy, for instance, is a safe and feasible approach for benign gallbladder disease. Its utility extends to more complicated biliary pathology, as it can be combined with common bile duct exploration to address complicated biliary pathology in a single setting, thereby showcasing its capability for complex benign biliary interventions. Further evidence from studies comparing robotic versus laparoscopic cholecystectomy for benign gallbladder disease, while sometimes noting increased operative time for the robotic approach, generally confirmed safety and no significant differences in complications or bile duct injury (34,70,71). Robotic management of a primary cholecystoduodenal fistula, a rare and complex benign biliary pathology, has also been successfully reported as a safe and favorable approach. This suggests the potential of robotic surgery as a preferred method, especially for patients anticipated to face significant laparoscopic morbidity due to the fistula's inherent complexity (72). These expansions into complex benign HPB conditions underscore the versatile advantages of the robotic platform, leveraging its precision and advanced visualization for delicate anatomical situations that might otherwise require open surgery.

The application of robotic liver resection also extends to cases complicated by challenging patient factors, such as cirrhosis or a history of prior abdominal surgeries. For cirrhotic patients, liver resection inherently presents increased challenges due to impaired synthetic liver function and a heightened risk of bleeding. Robotic liver resection offers identifiable advantages in these vulnerable patients, where enhanced visualization, precise dissection, and meticulous hemostasis are critically important to minimize trauma to the fragile liver parenchyma and preserve remnant liver function (73). The ability to perform more extensive or complex minimally invasive operations, including repeat resections in patients with extensive adhesions from previous abdominal surgeries, is a notable advantage of the robotic approach (74).

Despite these benefits, the high cost of robotic surgery remains a drawback that can limit its widespread application for benign liver diseases, particularly when clinical benefits do not clearly outweigh costs compared to established laparoscopic methods. More studies are continuously needed to definitively justify the broader introduction of robotic surgery for benign liver diseases and to precisely define the specific patient types that would most optimally benefit from its advanced capabilities (67).

3.4 Overcoming the Learning Curve and Expert Contributions

The adoption of robotic liver surgery, particularly for complex resections, inherently involves a recognized steep learning curve. This period of skill acquisition is a critical phase for any new surgical technology, as proficiency must be achieved without compromising patient safety. For robotic procedures in general, a recognized learning curve is associated, meaning dedicated practice and training are required for surgeons to achieve proficiency. Achieving consistently excellent clinical outcomes and ensuring optimal patient safety in HPB robotic procedures necessitated specific and extensive training in both highly specialized hepato-biliary surgery and broader general minimally invasive surgical techniques to effectively overcome this learning curve (21,46,47,66).

Expert contributions from pioneering surgeons and the establishment of high-volume centers were absolutely instrumental in meticulously defining and refining robotic surgical techniques, as well as consistently demonstrating the fundamental feasibility and safety of these increasingly advanced procedures (21,25). Their accumulated experience and willingness to innovate in uncharted surgical territory provided the initial roadmap for widespread adoption. For example, a multicenter randomized controlled trial comparing robotic pancreaticoduodenectomy (RPD) with open pancreaticoduodenectomy (OPD) explicitly noted that participating surgeons had already surpassed their individual learning curves of at least 40 RPD and 60 OPD procedures prior to their participation in the trial. This level of accumulated experience allowed the trial to effectively assess outcomes for proficient robotic surgeons, demonstrating that for surgeons who had passed the learning curve, RPD was safe and feasible, with the advantage of shorter postoperative length of hospital stay than OPD (75). Preliminary reports from other major pancreatic surgery series also showed encouraging results with morbidity and mortality comparable to open surgery, indicating the transferability of skills and experience across the HPB domain (63).

Consensus guidelines, such as those formulated by the ROBOT4HPB conference, represented a collaborative and multidisciplinary initiative to establish the first guidelines on the safety and indications of robotics in Hepato-Pancreato-Biliary (HPB) surgery. These guidelines supported the feasibility of robotics for most HPB procedures and its potential value in extending minimally invasive indications, emphasizing, however, the importance of expertise to ensure safety. The concept of expertise was defined broadly, encompassing requirements for credentialing HPB robotics at a given center. They also highlighted the need for prospective registries, including validated outcome metrics, for the forthcoming assessment of HPB robotics. The overall aim was to establish the first consensus guidelines on the safety and indications of robotics in HPB surgery, and to identify priorities for future research. These guidelines produced recommendations covering technology, training and expertise, outcome assessment, and liver and pancreatic procedures (76).

Advantages of a robotic approach to liver resection specifically include a shortened learning curve for surgeons when compared to laparoscopic approaches, facilitating a quicker path to proficiency. Furthermore, the robotic platform provided the ability to complete more extensive or complex minimally invasive operations than previously feasible with conventional laparoscopy (31). As surgeons become more skilled and robotic programs gain experience, patients are increasingly benefiting from this expanding technology. The continuous efforts to enhance surgical technique are necessary to overcome challenges such as longer operative times observed in early robotic procedures (77). The stepwise growth of robot-assisted surgery in the liver, in contrast to the rapid adoption of laparoscopic cholecystectomy, has allowed for a more structured identification of areas for improvement and a focus on combined efforts between engineers and surgeons. Despite an initial lack of early adoption by many hepatobiliary surgeons, robotic liver surgery continues to evolve and find its place within hepatobiliary surgery, with increasing evidence supporting its feasibility and safety in resections, including those of the posterior segments (22,32). Complex robotic liver resections are considered safe and feasible once the steep learning curve of the surgical team has plateaued (8). Standardized education and certification for future generations of surgeons considering robotic surgery is also crucial to ensure patient safety, as the use of robots in surgery continues to expand (33). Larger, prospective cohorts will also provide more definitive evidence of the benefits of robotic surgery.

3.5 Comparison with Laparoscopic Liver Resection: Early Perspectives

In the early stages of its development, robotic liver surgery was frequently evaluated through direct comparison with the more established laparoscopic liver resection to assess its relative advantages and disadvantages, and to define its precise role in the surgical armamentarium. While minimally invasive hepatic resection surgery, in general, including laparoscopic approaches, had already demonstrated decreased perioperative morbidity and shorter hospital stays in selected patients, conventional laparoscopic liver resection inherently suffered from limitations such as reduced freedom of movement within the abdominal cavity and a limited 2-dimensional view of the operative. The absence of haptic feedback and the limitations of rigid, linear instruments further constrained complex maneuvers, particularly in the highly vascular liver (21,31,77).

Robotic systems were perceived as a direct technological

advancement designed to address these fundamental shortcomings of laparoscopy. Robot-assisted laparoscopy, including its application in hepatobiliary surgery, provides substantial improvements in surgical handling. The distinct advantages inherently offered by this advanced technique include significantly improved dexterity, which translates into increased surgical precision, and the effective elimination of physiological tremor or fatigue. The use of robotic surgery for hepatic procedures originated from its technical potential to overcome several major technical limitations known from conventional laparoscopy. This allowed for the possibility of performing more extended liver resections (22,31).

Early comparative studies showed that using the robotic technique was associated with a decreased or at least equal amount of intraoperative blood loss compared to that of the conventional laparoscopic or open technique (22). Oncologic outcomes of robotic hepatectomy appeared to be equivalent to laparoscopic and open hepatectomy for appropriately selected patients (31). Robotic liver resection also offered more favorable postoperative patient recovery, and like laparoscopic hepatectomy, it could provide patients with more rapid recovery and a shorter hospital stay, which could help offset the substantial costs of robot acquisition and maintenance (22,31).

Despite these promising early results and demonstrated technical advantages, the added benefit of the robotic platform over conventional laparoscopy remained a matter of ongoing investigation. The overall available data from early reviews showed the noninferiority of the robotic system to conventional open and laparoscopic surgery. Some studies even suggested potential advantages for performing high-demanding procedures in a minimally invasive fashion using the robotic platform. However, the lack of large, multicenter, randomized controlled trials, directly comparing robotic liver surgery with open and laparoscopic surgery, precluded the possibility of reaching definitive conclusions regarding its superior value. Specific controversies continued to exist regarding robotic liver resection, despite its increasing application and perceived benefits due to technical advancements.

The overall data regarding robotic liver resection has been summarized, focusing on current indications and short-term and oncologic outcomes (8,9,22,29,54,78).

Recent advances in minimally invasive surgery, including both laparoscopic and robotic techniques, have notably changed the paradigm of surgical treatment for hepatobiliary diseases, offering advantages such as minimal wound extension for cosmetic effect, early postoperative recovery, and few postoperative complications (77). Early comparisons in other complex HPB procedures, such as robotic versus laparoscopic distal pancreatectomy (RDP vs. LDP), indicated that robotic surgery could overcome difficulties and technical limits of laparoscopic surgery due to improved surgical manipulation and better visualization. This often led to benefits like a significantly higher rate of spleen preservation, a lower rate of conversion to open surgery, and a shorter hospital stay for RDP, although it incurred a higher cost compared to LDP (79). While laparoscopic pancreatic resection had shown benefits over open approaches (e.g., less blood loss, shorter hospital stay, fewer wound complications) and oncologic non-inferiority, the advent of robotics further introduced potential advantages (80). Data on robotic pancreatic surgery showed a trend towards improving outcomes such as operative time, estimated blood loss, and length of stay, while still offering the benefits of minimally invasive surgery (33). For example, a multicenter, open-label randomized controlled trial comparing robotic pancreaticoduodenectomy (RPD) with open pancreaticoduodenectomy (OPD) showed that for surgeons who had passed the learning curve, RPD was safe and feasible, with the advantage of a shorter postoperative length of hospital stay than OPD. This trial found that postoperative length of hospital stay was significantly shorter in the RPD group compared to the OPD group (median 11.0 days vs. 13.5 days), with similar rates of 90-day mortality and severe complications (75). While RPD could be associated with slightly better overall survival, it also generally came with higher costs (81). These comparisons across HPB subfields continuously informed the evolving understanding of robotic liver surgery's distinct advantages and limitations in its pioneering years. The complexity of pancreatic procedures warrants them to be carried out in specialized centers, where short and long-term outcomes seem to be similar to the ones achieved in open surgery (63). Minimally invasive approaches, including both laparoscopic and robot-assisted techniques, are being performed more frequently to remove pancreatic cancers. Perioperative care has been refined by MIS, optimized surgical techniques, and structured complication management, contributing to improving outcomes (82). These advancements and early comparisons solidified the foundation for the continued expansion of robotic liver surgery.

Chapter 4: Technological Advancements Driving Robotic Hepatic Expansion

The surgical theater, a domain historically defined by the meticulous skill of human hands, has witnessed an unparalleled transformation over the past few decades. At the heart of this revolution lies the integration of robotic surgical systems, a progression that has particularly profound implications for the intricate landscape of Hepato-Pancreato-Biliary (HPB) surgery. This profound shift was never a singular event, nor a mere conceptual leap; rather, it has been inextricably linked to, and powerfully propelled by, a continuous and accelerating stream of sophisticated technological advancements. These groundbreaking innovations systematically addressed the inherent limitations that had previously constrained conventional minimally invasive techniques, thereby significantly expanding the surgical capabilities of the robotic platform and enabling its increasing utility in intricate liver and pancreatic procedures, areas once considered too complex for anything but open approaches.

The journey of robot-assisted surgery in the liver has unfolded with a deliberate and calculated stepwise approach, a stark contrast to the almost frenzied, rapid adoption observed with simpler procedures like laparoscopic cholecystectomy. This controlled, methodical growth allowed for the precise identification of critical areas ripe for improvement, many of which reside at the intricate nexus where advanced engineering principles meet precise medical practice. As robotic systems evolved from their rudimentary beginnings to increasingly sophisticated iterations, they brought forth a new era defined by profoundly enhanced instrumentation, vastly superior visualization modalities, and crucial ergonomic improvements for the operating surgeon. Collectively, these advancements have served as the relentless engine propelling the expansion of robotic hepatic surgery into realms previously considered daunting or even unapproachable by minimally invasive means. This chapter will illuminate these pivotal technological advancements that have not only achieved significant clinical presence but have, in essence, actively driven the very expansion of robotic hepatic surgery to its current, cutting-edge state.

4.1 Enhanced Instrumentation and Visualization

At the core of the robotic revolution in hepatic surgery lies the relentless pursuit of perfection in surgical tools and the visual clarity with which the surgeon navigates the operative field. A true cornerstone of the technological advancements driving robotic hepatic expansion has been the significant and continuous enhancement of both surgical instrumentation and the visualization systems available to the surgeon.

Revolutionary Instrumentation: Traditional laparoscopic instruments, while hailed as revolutionary in their time for enabling minimally invasive access, often presented a fundamental limitation: their rigid, linear design severely restricted dexterity due to inherently limited degrees of freedom. This fundamental design constraint rendered many highly intricate surgical tasks, particularly those demanding fine manipulation or complex suturing, extremely challenging to perform effectively. Robotic surgery was specifically developed with the explicit aim to directly address and elegantly overcome these very issues, providing a transformative platform that could transcend the limitations of conventional laparoscopic tools (10,22,62).

Key improvements in instrumentation are epitomized by the development of articulated instruments, universally recognized and frequently referred to as "endo-wrists". These advanced instruments are meticulously designed with a groundbreaking capability: they faithfully mimic the natural dexterity, articulation, and expansive seven degrees of freedom characteristic of the human hand and wrist (6,23,25). This unparalleled articulation provides surgeons with highly operable tools, offering exceptional maneuverability even within the most confined anatomical spaces—a feature particularly advantageous in the complex and often deep abdominal cavity, where delicate HPB procedures are routinely performed. Furthermore, the ongoing development of multi-degree-of-freedom (multi-DOF) wrist mechanisms represents a continuous commitment in the field to combine unparalleled precision with significantly improved surgical accessibility (23). Beyond dexterity, the robotic system inherently incorporates sophisticated tremor-filtering technology, which effectively dampens and eliminates natural physiological hand tremors, and advanced motion scaling functions. These functionalities precisely translate larger, often less precise, hand movements from the surgeon's console into smaller, more stable, and exquisitely precise instrument movements within the patient's body, thereby significantly enhancing overall surgical precision (4,10). Such mechanical advantages are not merely conveniences; they are crucial for performing delicate dissections and achieving precise suturing, maneuvers that are commonplace and critical in HPB surgery, contributing to safer and more effective interventions (63).

Unprecedented Visualization: In parallel with the evolution of instrumentation, significant and continuous improvements in visualization capabilities have proven absolutely critical in actively driving the expansion of robotic hepatic surgery. Early laparoscopic systems, while offering a less invasive window into the body, were notably limited by a two-dimensional (2D) monoscopic visual field, which profoundly compromised the surgeon's depth perception—a truly critical element for precise dissection, accurate tissue manipulation, and navigating the complex, three-dimensional anatomy of a vascular organ like the liver. Robotic platforms directly and fundamentally addressed this visual limitation by providing a high-resolution, three-dimensional (3D) magnified field of view. This advanced stereoscopic visualization capability dramatically improves depth perception, offering a distinct and profound advantage when compared to the traditional 2D monoscopic vision typically available in early laparoscopic systems (4,6,10). The undeniable significance of 3D vision is such that it has led to a broader professional consensus recommending its routine use in general laparoscopy as a robust means to potentially reduce overall operative time (24). The da Vinci system, for instance, exemplifies this advancement by providing an excellent field of view via a high-definition three-dimensional monitor (4).

Beyond the foundational 3D view, advanced imaging modalities have been seamlessly and progressively integrated into robotic platforms, providing crucial intraoperative advantages that are particularly beneficial for the complexities of HPB surgery. The critical incorporation of indocyanine green (ICG) fluorescence imaging has proven to be a highly valuable intraoperative tool. ICG fluorescence is particularly valuable for the precise and real-time recognition of complex vascular and biliary anatomy during hepatobiliary surgery, thereby significantly enhancing both surgical safety and accuracy (25,83). This supplementary technology aids in providing an expanded field of vision and crucial anatomical landmarks that might otherwise be obscured. Such fluorescence-guided technologies, including near-infrared fluorescence (NIRF), have proven valuable for various applications, helping to identify critical structures and minimize complications. These collective and synergistic technological leaps directly and effectively addressed the numerous technical hurdles inherent in traditional laparoscopic approaches, thereby significantly extending the viable and safe options for minimally invasive surgery to a broader spectrum of complex general surgical procedures, particularly those previously deemed too challenging and requiring intricate movements or access to anatomically difficult areas.

4.2 Haptic Technology and Ergonomics

The evolution of robotic platforms has been profoundly influenced not only by advances in core instrumentation and visualization but also by continuous improvements in the sensory feedback provided to the surgeon and the physical comfort of the operating environment. These advancements in haptic (tactile) technology and ergonomics are crucial for enhancing the surgeon's overall experience and, ultimately, optimizing patient outcomes.

The Quest for Haptic Technology: A significant and universally recognized limitation of early robotic systems, which remains an active area of research and development, was the complete absence of haptic (tactile) feedback. This fundamental lack of tactile sensation posed formidable technical hurdles for executing highly intricate maneuvers, particularly in delicate and highly vascular environments such as the hepatic milieu, where precise tissue handling, discerning tissue planes, and assessing tension feedback are absolutely critical. The robotic platform initially remained limited by this profound lack of haptic feedback, as well as a paucity of dedicated parenchymal transection devices, both of which are crucial for safe and effective liver surgery. Despite these persistent challenges, the pursuit of more intuitive and responsive surgical systems that can provide some form of haptic feedback continues to drive relentless innovation, actively aiming to bridge the critical sensory gap between robotic and traditional open surgery's tactile experience. Promisingly, some newer platforms now entering or expanding clinical use, such as the Senhance Surgical System, have already successfully integrated haptic feedback, contributing not only to improved ergonomics but also to a more intuitive and responsive surgical feel (84).

Ergonomics and Enhanced Surgeon Comfort: Concurrently with these technical pursuits, enhanced ergonomics and optimization of surgeon comfort have emerged as pivotal advancements, significantly contributing to the broader adoption and improved performance of robotic platforms in complex cases. Conventional laparoscopy, despite its minimally invasive benefits, could be physically demanding for surgeons due to the awkward postures, static and often uncomfortable positions, and prolonged periods of standing required, frequently leading to significant physical strain, chronic fatigue, and various musculoskeletal discomforts. Robotic systems, by striking contrast, offer substantial and undeniable ergonomic improvements. The surgeon operates from a comfortable, seated position at a console, which profoundly mitigates physical strain and significantly reduces the onset of fatigue, particularly crucial during long and intricate surgical procedures (1,10,85,86). This improved ergonomic comfort is not merely about convenience; it directly helps maintain surgeon focus, precision, and endurance over extended operative times, thereby safeguarding surgical performance (1,4). Indeed, the enhanced ergonomics, synergistically combined with improved dexterity and precision, allow robotic surgery to effectively augment the physical capabilities of surgeons, thereby overcoming inherent human physiological limitations such as involuntary physiological tremor and the insidious onset of fatigue. The da Vinci Xi, for instance, exemplifies this by offering a superb field of view and highly operable forceps, complemented by motion scale functions, and tremor-filtered articulated functions, all meticulously designed to contribute to a superior ergonomic experience for the surgeon (4). Studies have consistently demonstrated that robotics confers superior ergonomic benefits and a reduced workload compared to laparoscopy, benefiting both experienced surgeons and trainees alike (86). Self-reported discomfort was also notably lower in robotic procedures when compared to both laparoscopy and traditional open surgery (86). This continuous and unwavering emphasis on surgeon well-being is undeniably vital for the sustainable and highly effective integration of complex robotic technologies into surgical practice, particularly as procedures become progressively longer and more intricately demanding. Ergonomic interventions are crucial in both laparoscopic and robotic surgeries to enhance surgeon efficiency and well-being, emphasizing the need for ergonomic training and improved workstation setups (85,87).

4.3 Evolution of Robotic Platforms and New Technologies

The landscape of robotic surgery has experienced a dynamic and continuous evolution, extending significantly beyond the initial introduction of the da Vinci system. This progression has been marked by ongoing developments introducing novel designs, enhanced functionalities, and expanding capabilities that have already achieved significant clinical presence and thereby actively driven the expansion of robotic hepatic surgery to its current state. The focus here is firmly on platforms and technologies that are part of the established operative reality and their historical impact on expanding hepatic surgical indications.

The da Vinci Surgical System has, since its market introduction in 2000, undeniably dominated the surgical robot market, consistently demonstrating surgical feasibility across a myriad of procedures(6,8). However, the landscape of surgical robotics has begun to diversify rapidly, with multiple novel multi-port robotic surgical systems now actively being introduced into clinical practice. Examples of these newer, clinically available platforms include Micro Hand S, Senhance, Revo-i MSR-5000, KangDuo, Versius, and Hugo™ RAS (19). These contemporary systems often feature innovative modular designs, open or semi-open consoles designed for enhanced communication, smaller instruments to facilitate broader access, and are frequently developed with explicit aims of decreased cost, directly addressing some of the pervasive financial barriers to widespread adoption (77,88). This burgeoning development of alternative platforms signifies a crucial and important evolutionary phase in minimally invasive surgery, characterized by increasing competition and a robust, innovation-driven push to further expand surgical capabilities within the robotic surgery landscape (18).

- **Established Multi-Port Systems (e.g., da Vinci Xi and**

later iterations): The da Vinci platform itself has undergone a relentless and iterative process of continuous development since its initial inception, with the da Vinci Xi representing its advanced fourth generation (4). This ongoing evolution in robotic system design has consistently aimed to promote superior surgical performance and effectively reduce the physical and mental workload experienced by surgeons, solidifying its role in complex current procedures. These mature platforms have significantly expanded capabilities, including improved port placement flexibility and enhanced instrument reach, directly impacting the feasibility of more complex hepatic resections that are now routinely performed (22).

- **Clinically Present Alternative Multi-Port Systems:** The active introduction and growing utilization of systems like Senhance and Hugo™ RAS represent the current, diversifying state of robotic options available to surgeons. The Senhance Surgical System, for instance, allows for unique features such as infrared eye tracking and has integrated haptic feedback, complemented by an adjustable upright seat, all contributing to improved ergonomics and broader clinical utility(84). Similarly, the Hugo™ RAS system, with its distinctive open console and modular design, offers compelling advantages such as improved communication and enhanced ergonomics, along with increased flexibility for multi-quadrant surgeries, further expanding its current clinical applicability (89). These systems actively contribute to the current and expanding landscape of robotic platforms available for complex hepatic surgery.

- **Single-Port Robotic Systems with Current Clinical Application:** A significant evolutionary trend that has demonstrably entered widespread clinical practice and, by doing so, has substantially expanded the scope of minimally invasive surgery is the development of single-port robotic systems. The da Vinci single-port (SP) platform, for example, is a prime illustration, allowing the sophisticated insertion of three robotic instruments and an articulated scope through a single small incision. This innovative design explicitly aims to overcome the inherent limitations of both single-incision laparoscopic surgery and established multi-port robotic surgery, offering a more consolidated access point(90). While initially adopted widely in urological practice for both malignant and benign conditions, single-port robotic systems now demonstrably offer benefits in terms of improved cosmesis, better postoperative pain control, and decreased length of hospital stay in various applications (91,92). These advantages are also actively being explored and applied in HPB contexts, with robotic biliary surgery utilizing both multiport and single-port cholecystectomy techniques in current practice (71). The SHURUI single-port robotic system is another compelling example, demonstrating early clinical efficacy and safety in various urologic operations, further solidifying the current relevance of single-port designs (93). These single-port systems represent a critical development in contemporary minimally invasive surgery, offering tangible benefits in cost and pain control compared to traditional multi-port approaches (91).

- **Hybrid Approaches:** The continuous drive for innovation in current practice also extends to the development of hybrid approaches, which ingeniously combine robotic and traditional laparoscopic methods. This allows for greater flexibility and offers potential benefits in managing complex cases, representing a current refinement in surgical strategy (88).

These profound advancements in robotic platform design, ranging from the continuous refinement of multi-port systems to the significant emergence and current clinical application of single-port capabilities, collectively underscore the unyielding drive to push the boundaries of robotic surgery. They have already demonstrably facilitated the expansion of robotic procedures, particularly within the highly demanding fields like hepatic surgery, directly contributing to current clinical practices that offer greater precision, enhanced safety, and tangible patient benefit. Ultimately, further improvements in robot-assisted surgery in the years to come will continue to depend significantly on the combined and collaborative efforts of both engineers and surgeons.

Part III: Expanding Indications and Refinements in Robotic Liver Surgery

Chapter 5: Expanding the Operative Spectrum: Major Hepatectomies and Complex Cases

The application of robotic surgical platforms marked a pivotal and transformative moment in minimally invasive liver surgery, profoundly expanding its operative spectrum beyond the initial, simpler resections to encompass highly complex procedures, including major hepatectomies and the management of challenging tumor locations. This profound progression was a direct and necessary response to the inherent limitations that had previously constrained conventional laparoscopic techniques. Despite their initial benefits, traditional laparoscopic methods often struggled significantly with providing the requisite precision, optimal control, and comprehensive visualization demanded for intricate hepatic interventions. These persistent technical constraints included rigid instruments, a two-dimensional (2D) visual field compromising depth perception, and a notable absence of haptic (tactile) feedback, posing considerable technical hurdles for meticulous parenchymal transection, precise vascular control, and delicate intracorporeal suturing within the sensitive hepatic milieu (10). It was against this backdrop of persistent surgical challenges that robotic surgery emerged, promising to elevate precision and patient safety, particularly for demanding liver operations. The unique and advanced advantages inherently offered by robotic systems provided a compelling new pathway to safely and effectively address these exceedingly demanding surgical scenarios, thereby transforming the landscape of liver surgery.

The growth of robot-assisted surgery in the liver has unfolded as a deliberate stepwise approach, which is notably different from the rapid and widespread adoption (often described as a "frenzy") observed with the introduction of laparoscopic cholecystectomy. This controlled, stepwise growth allowed for the identification of critical areas for improvement, many of which reside at the intricate nexus of advanced engineering and precise medical practice. Further improvements in robot-assisted surgery, therefore, depend significantly on the combined efforts of both engineers and surgeons. This chapter will meticulously detail how robotic platforms have expanded the operative spectrum, enabling major and anatomic liver resections, addressing centrally located and hilar tumors, refining the management of complex vascular and biliary structures, and facilitating resections in challenging patient scenarios.

5.1 Robotic Major and Anatomic Liver Resections

The performance of robotic major hepatectomy, rigorously defined as the resection of three or more liver segments, represents a profoundly significant expansion of minimally invasive capabilities within the domain of liver surgery (64). This advanced procedure showcases the evolution of robotic applications from simpler tasks to highly intricate anatomical resections, pushing the boundaries of what is achievable through minimally invasive means.

Early systematic reviews, dedicated to the evaluation of robot-assisted major hepatectomy, meticulously analyzed initial pioneering cohorts of patients, thereby demonstrating the fundamental feasibility and potential safety of these highly complex surgical procedures. For instance, a systematic review published in 2014 provided a comprehensive analysis of 68 robotic major hepatectomies, encompassing both right (38 cases) and left (30 cases) hepatectomies, reflecting the primary forms of major liver resections undertaken. Crucially, this pioneering series reported no mortalities, which served as a vital early indicator of the safety profile of robotic major hepatectomy. The conversion rate to open surgery, a key metric for minimally invasive procedures, was notably low in these early major resections, recorded at 5.2% for right hepatectomies and 3.3% for left hepatectomies. These compelling early findings provided strong support for the assertion that major hepatectomy could indeed be performed effectively under robotic assistance, laying the groundwork for broader adoption (64).

While early operative times for these procedures averaged 418.6 minutes and intraoperative blood loss was approximately 411.4 mL, these metrics were considered acceptable given the complexity of the surgeries. Only a small percentage of patients (6.3%) required blood transfusions, and the overall postoperative complication rate stood at 26.9%. This foundational work underscored that while further experience was acknowledged as necessary before drawing final definitive conclusions, the initial data robustly supported the feasibility of robotic major hepatectomy (64). Robot-assisted hepatobiliary surgery, which includes major and extended hepatectomies, has been steadily growing in recent years and represents a viable alternative to open and laparoscopic approaches in selected patients (25).

Beyond the broad category of major resections, robotic surgery has enabled a significantly more precise approach to anatomic liver resections. This includes highly detailed procedures such as segmentectomies and sectionectomies, which demand an intricate understanding and execution of liver anatomy. Anatomical liver resection with Glissonean pedicle isolation is widely acknowledged and approved as an absolutely essential procedure for ensuring both surgical safety and oncological curability. In particular, the extrahepatic Glissonean pedicle isolation, performed without causing parenchymal destruction, is considered an ideal surgical maneuver. However, the standardization of this precise surgical technique has historically been challenging due to a perceived lack of comprehensive anatomical understanding. To address this, a novel comprehensive surgical anatomy of the liver, meticulously based on Laennec's capsule, has been proposed. This new anatomical framework provides a crucial theoretical background for the precise extrahepatic Glissonean pedicle isolation. Laennec's capsule is described as the proper membrane that not only covers the entire surface of the liver, including the bare area, but also intimately surrounds the intrahepatic Glissonean pedicles. Consequently, a distinct anatomical gap exists between the Glissonean pedicle and Laennec's capsule. This gap can be safely accessed extrahepatically, thereby allowing for the systematic isolation of the extrahepatic Glissonean pedicle without causing undesirable parenchymal destruction (65). This novel anatomical insight, applicable to both laparoscopic and robotic liver resection, is poised to significantly contribute to the standardization of surgical techniques for systematic extrahepatic Glissonean pedicle isolation in anatomical liver resection. Ultimately, this leads to bringing innovative changes in hepatobiliary surgery, thus spreading safer and more curable liver resections (65).

The inherent technical advantages of robotic systems, such as the enhanced dexterity provided by EndoWrist instruments and improved three-dimensional (3D) visualization, are particularly advantageous for these precise anatomical dissections. These technical benefits allow for better control during selective bleeding control, micro suturing, and fine dissection, which are critical in complex anatomic resections. The expansion of the operative spectrum in liver surgery to include not only major resections but also highly precise anatomic resections was a direct consequence of robotic capabilities that systematically addressed and overcame the limitations inherent in conventional laparoscopy, such as restricted freedom of movement and a 2D visual. Robotic surgery provides a platform that profoundly improves surgical handling. It offers distinct advantages such as significantly improved dexterity, which directly translates into a measurable increase in surgical precision, and the effective elimination of physiological tremor and a significant reduction in surgeon fatigue, both crucial factors during long and demanding liver operations. These enhanced capabilities were instrumental in facilitating the performance of more extended and technically challenging liver resections.

For example, robotic platforms demonstrate a particular efficacy in addressing lesions in the posterior-superior segments, which are notoriously difficult to access and resect effectively using traditional laparoscopic techniques (22). A meta-analysis comparing robotic versus laparoscopic liver resection for difficult posterosuperior segments showed that robotic liver resection was associated with less estimated blood loss, fewer blood transfusions, and shorter operative time, with no differences in postoperative morbidity, mortality, or R1 resection rates (69). This highlights the specific benefits of robotics for these anatomically demanding locations. The increasing application of robotic liver resection has consistently shown benefits in various aspects, directly attributable to the continuous technical advancement of the robotic surgical system (54).

5.2 Robotic Resection for Centrally Located and Hilar Tumors

The surgical resection of centrally located liver tumors and those intimately situated at the hepatic hilum represents one of the most formidable and technically demanding frontiers in all of liver surgery, demanding extreme precision due to the tumors' direct proximity to, and often involvement of, major vascular and biliary structures. Robotic surgery has shown particular and growing promise in expanding the range of minimally invasive options available for these exceedingly complex cases.

While early robotic liver resections aimed to establish general feasibility and safety, the distinctive technological advantages of the robotic platform, such as enhanced visualization and articulated instruments, are especially attractive and beneficial for navigating these highly demanding and anatomically intricate surgical landscapes. The ability to achieve exquisitely precise dissection and meticulous control around critical central structures is absolutely paramount for successful outcomes in these procedures.

Robotic systems inherently offer a high-resolution, three-dimensional (3D) magnified view of the surgical site. This significantly enhances the surgeon's ability to precisely identify, delineate, and safely navigate the complex vascular and biliary anatomy within the central liver, including those structures deeply embedded within the parenchyma or intricately located at the hepatic hilum. This improved depth perception is vital for accurately differentiating between arterial, portal venous, and hepatic venous structures, as well as the fine-branching bile ducts, all of which are tightly packed in the central liver and hilar regions. The use of 3D visualization technology is crucial for enhancing surgical accuracy in liver tumors, allowing for precise preoperative planning and intraoperative guidance.

The articulated endo-wristed instruments of robotic systems provide unparalleled dexterity and an expansive range of motion for manipulating and ligating vascular structures and performing fine, meticulous dissections around the biliary confluence. This enhanced precision allows for highly selective bleeding control, thereby minimizing overall blood loss during parenchymal transection—a consistently crucial factor in maintaining patient stability during liver surgery. The computer filtration of the surgeon's movements, a core robotic feature, further contributes to maintaining a remarkably stable operative field, thereby significantly reducing the risk of iatrogenic injury to vital structures during intricate maneuvers performed near the portal triad or major hepatic vein. This stability is especially critical for centrally located tumors where the risk of major vascular injury is high.

Robotic liver surgery has been shown to be feasible and safe in resections of the posterior segments (22), and specifically for the caudate lobe, which is deeply located and has complex vascular relationships, robotic resection demonstrates feasibility and safety with overall good outcomes (68). Robotic surgery has also demonstrated its ability to effectively handle major vascular anastomoses in other fields like renal and lung transplantation, and portal vein reconstruction, which are routinely performed with robotic assistance(94). These principles extend to robotic management of complex biliary pathology such as cholecystoduodenal fistula, suggesting the potential for robotic surgery as a preferred approach in cases anticipated to face significant laparoscopic morbidity due to complexity (72).

For pancreatic surgery, which frequently shares similar complexities with centrally located liver resections, the robotic platform has demonstrably enabled surgeons to perform procedures requiring intricate dissection along major abdominal vessels and delicate reconstruction involving biliary, pancreatic, and enteric anastomoses. Early reports from major robotic-assisted pancreatic surgery series, while not directly liver-focused, provided encouraging results with morbidity and mortality comparable to open surgery, indicating the transferability of skills and principles across the HPB domain (63). This experience in performing complex pancreatic resections, such as robotic central pancreatectomy for benign or low-grade tumors, further supports the expanding application of robotics to centrally located liver lesions, leveraging analogous surgical skills and technological advantages (95). These complex pancreatic procedures are often carried out in specialized centers, where accumulated expertise allows for short and long-term outcomes that appear to be similar to those achieved with open surgery (63). The specific benefits of robotics, including improved surgical manipulation and better visualization, were highlighted in meta-analyses comparing robotic versus laparoscopic distal pancreatectomy, where robotics showed advantages like higher spleen preservation and lower conversion rates (79). Such detailed benefits in neighboring HPB fields reinforce the rationale for applying robotics to equally challenging liver resections. Robotic pancreaticoduodenectomy (RPD) has shown benefits, including shorter length of hospital stay and fewer complications compared to open pancreaticoduodenectomy (OPD), with comparable oncological outcomes for surgeons who have passed the learning curve (75,96). This experience further underpins the capabilities for complex tumor resections within the HPB domain.

5.3 Management of Vascular Structures and Biliary Confluence

Effective and precise management of the liver's intricate vascular structures and the delicate biliary confluence is fundamentally critical for safe and successful hepatic surgery, particularly in complex cases involving major resections or centrally located tumors. Robotic surgery provides distinct and compelling advantages that significantly aid in these paramount aspects of liver intervention.

The three-dimensional (3D) magnified visualization inherently offered by robotic systems profoundly enhances the surgeon's ability to precisely identify, delineate, and meticulously navigate the complex vascular and biliary anatomy within the liver. This includes structures that are deeply embedded within the hepatic parenchyma or intricately located at the hepatic hilum. This dramatically improved depth perception is vital for accurately differentiating between the various components of the hepatic pedicle—including arterial, portal venous, and hepatic venous structures—as well as the fine branching bile ducts, all of which are tightly packed in the central liver and hilar regions. This detailed visualization is particularly important in ensuring minimal blood loss, a key benefit associated with robotic procedures.

The articulated endo-wristed instruments characteristic of robotic systems provide unparalleled dexterity and an expansive range of motion. This allows for highly precise manipulation and ligation of vascular structures and the performance of extremely fine, meticulous dissections around the delicate biliary confluence. This enhanced precision directly facilitates selective bleeding control, thereby significantly minimizing overall blood loss during parenchymal transection—a consistently crucial factor in maintaining patient stability and reducing morbidity during liver surgery. The computer filtration of surgeons' movements, a core robotic feature, further contributes to maintaining a remarkably stable operative field, thereby significantly reducing the risk of iatrogenic injury to vital structures during intricate maneuvers performed near the portal triad or major hepatic veins (22,63). This stability is particularly beneficial when dealing with highly friable hepatic tissue and large, easily injured vessels.

A profoundly significant technological advancement in this domain is the widespread adoption and integration of indocyanine green (ICG) fluorescence imaging. Seamlessly integrated into many modern robotic platforms, ICG fluorescence provides real-time, enhanced visualization of both vascular and biliary anatomy. This innovative imaging modality significantly aids in the precise recognition of structures that might otherwise be difficult to distinguish under standard white light, especially in complex cases, in livers with underlying pathology like cirrhosis, or when dealing with distorted anatomy (25,83). This can, for instance, assist in clearly identifying the demarcation of liver segments or the precise course of bile ducts, thereby substantially reducing the risk of bile leak or unintended vascular compromise. The development of systems for intraoperative ultrasound-guided robotic surgical procedures (RIOUS) further enhances visualization by allowing surgeons to "see through" parenchyma and into vascular structures, providing thorough assessment without additional radiation, leveraging the ergonomics and precision of robotic instruments (97). This capability is gaining relevance in general surgery fields including liver, pancreas, spleen, gallbladder/bile duct, vascular, and rectal surgery for locating tumors and defining resection margins. It overcomes limitations of restricted angulation and access within the abdominal cavity.

Furthermore, anatomical understanding plays a paramount role in managing these structures effectively. Systematic extrahepatic Glissonean pedicle isolation, an anatomical technique considered essential for safe and curable liver resection, can be significantly standardized and facilitated by insights from a novel comprehensive surgical anatomy based on Laennec's capsule. This technique, applicable to both laparoscopic and robotic liver resection, aids in systematically isolating the pedicle without parenchymal destruction, which is critical for precise management of vascular inflows to specific liver segments (65). The ability to perform complex reconstructions of the biliary tree during robotic cholecystectomy or other biliary procedures also explicitly underscores the platform's advanced capabilities in managing delicate HPB anatomy, extending to scenarios requiring complex biliary reconstruction. The use of robotic surgery for gallbladder cancer has demonstrated effectiveness as it can be combined with common bile duct exploration to address complicated pathology in a single setting (71).

5.4 Robotic Liver Resection in Complex Patient Scenarios

Robotic liver surgery has progressively and strategically expanded its indications to encompass a wide array of complex patient scenarios, where the inherent benefits of a minimally invasive approach can significantly impact overall patient outcomes, even in the presence of challenging confounding factors. This expansion notably includes patients with underlying diffuse liver conditions, such as cirrhosis, or those who necessitate repeat resections due to recurrent disease (66). Minimally invasive surgery (MIS), in general, for complex conditions like advanced renal cell carcinoma, has shown promise in improving perioperative outcomes without compromising oncologic control in properly selected patients, demonstrating a broader principle applicable to liver surgery (98).

For cirrhotic patients, liver resection inherently presents increased challenges due to impaired synthetic liver function, a heightened risk of bleeding from portal hypertension, and a generally higher propensity for postoperative liver failure. Robotic liver resection offers identifiable and distinct advantages for these vulnerable patients, where enhanced visualization, precise dissection, and meticulous hemostasis become even more critically important to minimize trauma to the fragile liver parenchyma and preserve remnant liver function. The robotic system's ability to achieve accurate and controlled hemostasis, coupled with its capacity for fine suturing with robotic instruments, can be profoundly beneficial in reducing the risk of complications such as blood loss and bile leaks in this vulnerable patient population (22). Robot-assisted major hepatectomy has been performed for malignant and benign tumors, with outcomes like low blood loss showing its potential in complex cases (64).

Robotic surgery has also demonstrated considerable promise and utility for patients undergoing repeat resections. In these cases, prior abdominal surgeries or previous liver resections can often lead to extensive and dense adhesions, as well as distorted anatomical planes, rendering subsequent operations exceptionally technically challenging and increasing the risk of iatrogenic injury. The robotic platform's articulated instruments and stable 3D visualization can significantly facilitate safe dissection through adhesions and help surgeons navigate altered anatomical planes with enhanced precision (22,26,99). The ability to perform more extensive or complex minimally invasive operations, including repeat resections, is a notable and compelling advantage of the robotic approach (31). The use of robotic surgery for lesions in the posterior-superior segments of the liver, which are notoriously difficult to access laparoscopically, highlights its utility in overcoming anatomical challenges. Specifically, robotic caudate lobectomy is considered feasible and safe despite the deep anatomic location of this segment and its relationships with major vessels, demonstrating good postoperative outcomes (68). A meta-analysis confirmed that robotic liver resection for difficult posterosuperior segments was associated with less estimated blood loss, fewer blood transfusions, and shorter operative time, with comparable morbidity and mortality to laparoscopic approaches (69).

Beyond these intrinsic liver conditions and repeat procedures, robotic surgery has further demonstrated its broad utility in other complex patient scenarios within the wider context of minimally invasive surgery for abdominal pathologies. The increasing adoption of minimally invasive pancreatectomy, despite its inherent challenges in consistently maintaining high-quality oncologic resection, demonstrates the continuous push to apply MIS to complex abdominal pathologies. Minimally invasive surgery for early-stage pancreatic cancer has yielded promising results regarding postoperative recovery and oncologic outcomes (82). Robotic pancreaticoduodenectomy (RPD), a highly complex procedure, has shown advantages such as shorter postoperative length of hospital stay and fewer complications compared to open pancreaticoduodenectomy (OPD), with comparable oncological outcomes for surgeons who have passed the learning curve (75,96). This highlights the potential of robotics to safely manage complex oncological cases with improved patient recovery. Robotic central pancreatectomy, for instance, showed low perioperative mortality despite high morbidity and pancreatic fistula rates, demonstrating feasibility in complex resections for benign/low-grade tumors (95).

Even the evolution of organ transplantation is becoming influenced by the adoption of minimally invasive techniques, transitioning from laparoscopic to robotic methods. Robotic surgery has emerged as a significant advancement in this field, providing superior precision and outcomes compared with traditional approaches. Studies reveal lower morbidity with robotic donor nephrectomy, recipient kidney transplant, and, importantly, robotic donor hepatectomy (100). Anesthetic considerations for robotic liver transplantation, while presenting unique challenges due to patient positioning and pneumoperitoneum, are manageable with thorough understanding and planning, requiring a deep understanding of liver disease, liver transplant surgery, and the various implications of robotic surgery to ensure optimal patient outcomes (101). The advantages of robotic liver surgery, such as improved 3D vision, enhanced dexterity, and the elimination of tremors, consistently contribute to less postoperative pain, less intraoperative blood loss, and a quicker return to normal activity, all of which are profoundly beneficial for complex and vulnerable patients (78,102).

These extensive expansions of robotic capabilities across various complex abdominal and HPB scenarios powerfully underscore its growing and indispensable role in safely managing the most demanding patient cases, extending the benefits of minimally invasive surgery to a broader population, including those with anatomical variations or prior surgical history. The increasing utilization of robotic surgery in surgical oncology, including HPB malignancies, reinforces its growing role as a powerful tool with promising short-term outcomes.

Chapter 6: Robotic Liver Surgery for Malignancy: Oncological Outcomes

The application of robotic surgical systems has profoundly expanded the capabilities of minimally invasive surgery, extending its reach to increasingly complex oncological procedures within the Hepato-Pancreato-Biliary (HPB) domain. While the initial years of robotic surgery focused on establishing feasibility and safety in general abdominal procedures, the inherent technical advantages of the robotic platform—including enhanced dexterity, superior three-dimensional (3D) visualization, and tremor filtration—made it an attractive tool for intricate cancer resections where precision is paramount. This chapter meticulously examines the role of robotic surgery in treating primary liver cancers and colorectal liver metastases, delving into the critical aspects of oncological clearance, lymphadenectomy, and long-term outcomes, thereby assessing its true value in the surgical management of hepatic malignancies. Robotic surgery has rapidly evolved, becoming particularly attractive as an alternative minimally invasive approach in liver surgery due to improvements in visualization and articulated instruments. Despite the lack of early adoption by many hepatobiliary surgeons, robotic liver surgery continues to evolve and find its place within hepatobiliary surgery. The use of robotic surgery for hepatic procedures originated because of the technical potential to overcome several major technical limitations known from conventional laparoscopy.

6.1 Robotic Resection for Primary Liver Cancers (HCC, Cholangiocarcinoma)

The surgical management of primary liver cancers, notably Hepatocellular Carcinoma (HCC) and Cholangiocarcinoma (CCA), demands extensive liver resection with a focus on oncological radicality while preserving sufficient liver tissue. Robotic liver resection (RLR) has increasingly been applied in recent years, demonstrating benefits owing to the technical advancements of robotic surgical systems. The increasing global utilization of robotic surgery for various procedures includes its robust application in surgical oncology, where it serves as a powerful tool for treating gastrointestinal, hepato-pancreatico-biliary, colorectal, endocrine, and soft tissue malignancies. While long-term outcomes are still emerging, short-term outcomes in robotic cancer surgery have shown promise.

For Hepatocellular Carcinoma (HCC), surgical resection remains a critical treatment modality, particularly for improving prognosis. The evolving landscape of HCC management includes the emerging role of robotic surgery as a technique that enhances surgical precision. This is facilitated by advanced technologies such as three-dimensional simulation and intraoperative navigation systems, which contribute to improved surgical accuracy and optimized surgical planning. Robot-assisted hepatic surgery in malignancy has been shown to be feasible and safe in resections, including those of the posterior-superior segments, which are technically challenging anatomical locations for minimally invasive approaches (22,32). Oncologic outcomes of robotic hepatectomy for appropriately selected patients appear to be equivalent to those achieved with laparoscopic and open hepatectomy (22,31,66). Studies consistently indicate that robotic techniques are associated with a decreased or at least equal amount of intraoperative blood loss compared to conventional laparoscopic or open techniques. The capacity to perform more extended liver resections in a minimally invasive fashion is a significant advantage of robotics, allowing for the treatment of larger or more complex HCCs. Minimally invasive methods for HCC, which are among the most common indications for surgery, can be safely applied in high-volume centers and by experienced surgeons (103). A multicenter propensity-score matched analysis compared robotic liver resection (RLR) with laparoscopic liver resection (LLR) for hepatocellular carcinoma (HCC) in 647 patients from 12 centers. The study aimed to investigate the benefits of RLR over LLR for HCC, considering perioperative and oncologic outcomes. After matching for various patient and tumor characteristics, RLR showed several significant perioperative advantages: wider surgical margins (median: 10 vs 5 mm, $p = 0.002$), a higher prevalence of R0 resection (98.9% vs 93.1%, $p = 0.037$), a lower conversion rate to open surgery (2.1% vs

8.5%, p = 0.039), and a shorter hospital stay (median: 4 vs 5 days, p = 0.025). There was no significant difference in the postoperative complication rate between the two groups. Regarding oncological outcomes, overall survival (OS) was similar between RLR and LLR cohorts (5-year OS: 68.7% vs 65.0%, p = 0.82). However, a notable finding was the significantly better recurrence-free survival (RFS) in the RLR cohort (5-year RFS: 46.8% vs 24.0%, p = 0.04). The study concluded that RLR for HCC offers significantly better perioperative outcomes, including wider resection margins associated with improved RFS, as well as a lower conversion rate and shorter hospital stay, although the latter may be influenced by the multi-institutional nature of the study (104).

For Cholangiocarcinoma, particularly perihilar cholangiocarcinoma (pCCA), open surgery remains the standard of care due to its complex nature, often requiring complex major hepatectomy with intricate biliary reconstruction. However, robotic liver surgery is emerging as a safe, minimally invasive technique with considerable potential for pCCA management. The first case of robotic-assisted liver resection with biliary reconstruction for pCCA was described by Giulianotti in 2010, marking a pioneering step in this highly challenging area of HPB surgery. Subsequent Western case series have presented preliminary data on the feasibility and repeatability of these procedures. For instance, a series of 6 major robotic liver resections with biliary reconstruction, including 4 for pCCA, demonstrated feasibility with a median operating time of 840 minutes and median blood loss of 700 ml. Notably, none of these patients experienced major complications, and negative biliary margins were achieved in three of the four pCCA cases, suggesting its potential for oncological radicality(105). The da Vinci platform's capability in multi-duct biliary reconstruction holds significant promise for pCCA surgery.

For hilar cholangiocarcinoma (HC), laparoscopic and robotic surgery have been summarized for safety and feasibility, with innovations in technology and gradual accumulation of surgical experience expected to improve outcomes. The pooled prevalence of R0 resection for HC in laparoscopic/robotic series was 80.1%

(85.9%/71.0% respectively), with a weighted mean operative time of 458.4 min and blood loss of 615.3 mL (106).

A network meta-analysis comparing robot-assisted (RA), laparoscopic-assisted (LA), and open surgery (OA) for cholangiocarcinoma aimed to evaluate the efficacy of these three surgical methods. The analysis of relevant literature, updated to September 1st, 2024, showed that RA surgery was superior to both LA and OA in several key outcomes. These superiorities included the length of R0 resection (achieving clear margins), complication rate, 30-day mortality, transfusion rate, lymph node metastasis rate, and hospital stay. However, when comparing operative time, the study found no significant difference among RA, LA, and OA surgery, with the relative effectiveness ranking from shortest to longest being open surgery, laparoscopic-assisted surgery, and robot-assisted surgery. The conclusion of the study affirmed that robot-assisted surgery is safe and feasible for treating cholangiocarcinoma, but it also emphasized the need for more clinical evidence to definitively confirm these findings (107).

Beyond these specific primary cancers, robotic surgery for gallbladder cancer (GBC) has also been evaluated. Both laparoscopic and robotic surgery are considered safe and effective approaches for the surgical management of GBC, with postoperative and survival outcomes comparable to open surgery. Minimally invasive approaches for GBC may lead to shorter hospitalization, less intraoperative blood loss, and fewer postoperative complications compared to open surgery. However, there was no obvious benefit of either MIS approach (laparoscopic versus robotic) over the other in this context, suggesting similar efficacy between the two minimally invasive methods(108). Other studies also support that robotic radical cholecystectomy offers certain potential advantages over open radical cholecystectomy for GBC, including reduced intraoperative blood loss, shorter hospital stay, and fewer overall complications, suggesting it might be an optimal choice for treating GBC (109). Compared to open surgery, robotic surgery for GBC had reduced intraoperative blood loss, shorter hospital stay, and fewer overall complications (109). Despite these promising results, robotic surgery for GBC has been limited to highly selected patients and is technically feasible in experienced surgeons, but improvements in techniques and instrumentation are still needed to further promote MIS in GBC treatment (110). Minimally invasive hepatobiliary surgery, encompassing both laparoscopic and robotic methods, shows better short-term results than open surgery in terms of blood loss, need for blood transfusion, length of intensive care unit and hospital stay, and postoperative major complication rate. These methods also demonstrate similar oncologic outcomes to open surgery (103).

6.2 Robotic Approaches for Colorectal Liver Metastases (CRLM)

Colorectal liver metastases (CRLM) represent a common and significant challenge in oncological surgery, often requiring highly complex resections to achieve curative intent. Robotic surgery has emerged as a promising minimally invasive approach for the management of CRLM, including simultaneous resections of primary colorectal cancer (CRC) and synchronous liver metastases (111,112).

Traditional open simultaneous resection of CRC and synchronous liver metastases is widely performed and offers a potential cure for eligible patients. However, the feasibility of robotic simultaneous resection of primary and secondary liver lesions had not been fully established as a treatment option for metastatic rectal cancer. A randomized controlled trial (RCT) comparing robotic-assisted simultaneous resection with open surgery in patients with rectal cancer and liver metastases demonstrated that the robotic group experienced fewer complications within 30 days after surgery (31.4% vs. 57.6%) and a faster recovery, including less blood loss (125.5 mL vs. 211.6 mL), faster bowel function recovery (63.7 h vs. 93.8 h), and shorter hospital stay (8.0 days vs. 10.7 days). Importantly, oncological outcomes, including the 3-year disease-free survival (DFS) rate (39.5% vs. 35.3%) and 3-year overall survival (OS) rate (76.7% vs. 72.9%), showed no statistically significant difference between the robotic and open groups (112).

This provides high-level evidence supporting robotic surgery for these complex simultaneous procedures, indicating it can match the oncological efficacy of open surgery while offering perioperative benefits.

Furthermore, a systematic review focusing specifically on robotic surgery for colorectal cancer liver metastases (CRCLM) resection highlighted that robotic-assisted surgery might be considered a technical upgrade option for a minimally invasive approach to CRCLM resections. This includes suitability even for simultaneous operations and challenging cases. The review of 262 patients who underwent robotic CRCLM resections reported a mean blood loss of 309.4 mL, a mean operative time of 250.5 minutes, and a mean length of hospital stay of 7.98 days. The overall postoperative mortality was notably low at 0.4%, and the overall morbidity rate was 37.0%, with Clavien-Dindo grade III-IV complications at 8.4%. The mean 3-year overall survival was 55.25%, and the mean 3-year disease-free survival was 37%. These results suggest that robotic-assisted surgery provides a safe and efficient minimally invasive approach for highly selected patients with CRCLM, always implemented within a multidisciplinary patient management context (111). These findings contribute to the growing body of evidence supporting the use of robotics in complex oncological settings.

The technical advantages of robotic systems, such as improved dexterity through endowristed instruments, enhanced three-dimensional visualization, and computer filtration of surgeon's movements, are particularly beneficial for the intricate dissections required in CRCLM resections, especially when combined with primary tumor resections. The ability to perform more extended liver resections in a minimally invasive fashion using robotics is crucial for CRLM, where tumor burden can be significant and often requires major resections. Overall, the accumulated evidence suggests that oncologic results after robotic liver resection for CRCLM are comparable to those achieved with open and laparoscopic approaches.

In the broader context of colorectal cancer surgery, robotic approaches have shown promising outcomes that influence the understanding of CRLM management. Robotic colorectal surgery, which allows better ergonomics, three-dimensional vision, and seven-degree freedom of movement, ensures fast recovery, fewer postoperative complications, and safe oncological resections (38). Studies have found that robotic rectal cancer surgery, for instance, leads to lower conversion rates and faster recovery of urogenital function compared to conventional laparoscopic surgery (113). Robotic surgery can also reduce the risk of circumferential resection margin positivity compared with conventional laparoscopic surgery in patients undergoing mesorectal excision for rectal cancer (114,115). This increased precision is particularly valuable in the narrow confines of the pelvis, and similar principles translate to complex liver resections.

6.3 Lymphadenectomy and Achieving Oncological Clearance

Achieving optimal oncological outcomes in liver and hepato-pancreato-biliary (HPB) surgery fundamentally relies on two distinct yet complementary principles: lymphadenectomy and R0 resection (oncological clearance). Lymphadenectomy pertains to the meticulous surgical removal and harvesting of regional lymph nodes, primarily within the liver hilum and surrounding peripancreatic-biliary regions (including around the head of the pancreas when involved in HPB malignancies like cholangiocarcinoma), for accurate disease staging and removal of potential microscopic metastases. In contrast, R0 resection, or oncological clearance, refers to the complete macroscopic and microscopic removal of the primary tumor, ensuring that no cancer cells are present at the surgical margins. Robotic surgery offers unique technical advantages that significantly facilitate both of these critical oncological goals, particularly in anatomically challenging HPB regions where major vessels and vital structures are in close proximity.

The enhanced precision, improved dexterity, and superior three-dimensional (3D) visualization provided by robotic systems are highly beneficial for performing meticulous lymph node dissections and achieving clear resection margins in complex HPB oncology. This precision is paramount when operating in deep, confined spaces, allowing for careful dissection around critical neurovascular structures while preserving vital tissue.

For primary liver cancers like Hepatocellular Carcinoma (HCC), while extensive lymphadenectomy is not always the primary focus, achieving R0 resection through precise parenchymal dissection is paramount for improving prognosis (116). Robotic liver resection for HCC offers significantly better perioperative outcomes, including achieving more R0 resection which is associated with improved RFS, as well as a lower conversion rate and shorter hospital stay, although the latter may be influenced by the multi-institutional nature of the study (104).

For Cholangiocarcinoma (CCA), particularly perihilar cholangiocarcinoma (pCCA) and hilar cholangiocarcinoma (HC), radical resection often necessitates extensive lymphadenectomy alongside complex major hepatectomy and intricate biliary reconstruction to achieve R0 resection and accurate staging due to its aggressive lymphatic spread (105). Robotic liver surgery is emerging as a safe, minimally invasive technique with considerable potential for CCA management. Early robotic series for hilar cholangiocarcinoma show a pooled prevalence of R0 resection at 71.0%, indicating its potential for radical resection in these challenging tumors, though further experience is needed (106). The da Vinci platform's capability in multi-duct biliary reconstruction, which is often crucial in these cases, holds significant promise for CCA surgery (105). The anatomical understanding and precise dissection facilitated by robotics, such as systematic extrahepatic Glissonean pedicle isolation, contribute directly to achieving clear margins and effective lymphadenectomy in liver resections.

For gallbladder cancer (GBC), achieving oncological clearance is critical, often involving extended liver resection and regional lymphadenectomy. Robotic radical cholecystectomy for GBC has shown potential advantages in achieving effective tumor resection and lymph node retrieval, along with benefits like reduced intraoperative blood loss and shorter hospital stay, contributing to safer oncological outcomes (108,109).

In the context of Colorectal Liver Metastases (CRLM), while the primary focus is often liver parenchymal resection, the overall oncological management often involves assessment of regional lymph nodes if the primary colorectal tumor is concurrently resected or if there is concern for nodal disease. Robotic approaches have demonstrated benefits in simultaneous resections of primary colorectal cancer and liver metastases, indicating their capacity to achieve oncological clearance in complex multi-site procedures (111,112). Robotic colorectal surgery (for the primary tumor) facilitates safe oncological resections, and principles learned from its use in difficult anatomical areas, such as the pelvis, where achieving clear margins and adequate lymph node dissection is challenging, translate to the precision required for liver resections. Robotic rectal cancer surgery, for instance, can reduce the risk of circumferential resection margin positivity in complex pelvic dissections, underscoring the precision that robotics can bring to oncological clearance (115).

For pancreatic malignancies, particularly in the head of the pancreas (which is intricately linked to the biliary system and liver via the HPB anatomy), achieving oncological clearance through pancreaticoduodenectomy (PD) is a highly complex procedure requiring extensive lymphadenectomy and R0 resection. Robotic-assisted pancreaticoduodenectomy (RPD) has shown promising oncological outcomes for pancreatic ductal adenocarcinoma (PDAC), including comparable or even superior margin status, higher lymph node harvest, and time to chemotherapy compared to open approaches(96). A multicenter randomized controlled trial of RPD versus OPD found similar rates of 90-day mortality and severe complications, with comparable oncological outcomes for surgeons who had passed the learning curve (75). This high-level evidence supports the oncological safety of robotic approaches in these complex HPB procedures that frequently involve extensive lymphadenectomy and meticulous clearance. The consistent ability to achieve a higher number of harvested lymph nodes in robotic pancreatic surgery signifies a thorough dissection, contributing directly to accurate staging and improved long-term outcomes (117,118).

Achieving negative resection margins (R0 resection) is a primary and non-negotiable goal in cancer surgery, as positive margins can lead to local recurrence and compromise long-term survival. For robotic liver resections, oncologic outcomes, including R0 resection rates, consistently appear to be equivalent to those of laparoscopic and open hepatectomy for appropriately selected patients (22,31,66). In the context of hilar cholangiocarcinoma, robotic surgery aims to achieve R0 resection, with a reported pooled prevalence of 71.0% in early robotic series, underscoring its potential for radical resection in these challenging tumors, though further experience is needed for clear conclusions (106). The importance of surgical expertise, formal guidelines (like those from ROBOT4HPB), and prospective registries for collecting validated outcome metrics is critical for assessing and ensuring oncological clearance in HPB robotics, pushing towards standardization and objective evaluation of results (76). The increasing utilization of robotic surgery in surgical oncology, including HPB malignancies, reinforces its growing role as a powerful tool with promising short-term outcomes, especially in achieving oncological clearance (7).

6.4 Long-Term Oncological Outcomes

The evaluation of robotic liver surgery for malignancy extends critically beyond short-term perioperative outcomes to meticulously assess long-term oncological results, which encompass crucial metrics such as recurrence rates, disease-free survival (DFS), and overall survival (OS). This comprehensive long-term assessment is absolutely paramount for definitively establishing the true value, widespread clinical utility, and sustainable adoption of any novel cancer treatment modality. While the evidence base for long-term outcomes specifically in robotic liver surgery is still actively maturing, accumulating data from various oncological procedures provides invaluable insights that inform the broader HPB context.

For primary liver cancers, including HCC, the evolving landscape of management increasingly integrates robotic surgery as a technique to enhance precision and potentially improve long-term outcomes. The emergence of robotic surgery, combined with other technical innovations like 3D simulation and intraoperative navigation systems, is integral to improving prognosis for HCC, though postoperative recurrence remains a significant and persistent challenge (116). While the increasing application of robotic liver resection has shown benefits due to technical advancements, some controversies still exist regarding its overall long-term role, indicating a continued need for more robust and mature long-term data. International consensus guidelines for robotic liver resection aim to update clinical recommendations and provide guidance to improve outcomes, including oncological ones, by consolidating available evidence and experts' opinions (54).

In the context of colorectal liver metastases (CRLM), robotic-assisted simultaneous resection of primary rectal cancer and synchronous liver metastases showed no statistically significant difference in 3-year disease-free survival (DFS) rate (39.5% vs. 35.3%) or 3-year overall survival (OS) rate (76.7% vs. 72.9%) compared to open surgery in a randomized controlled trial. This high-level evidence indicates comparable long-term oncological efficacy, despite the robotic approach offering benefits in short-term complications and recovery (112). Similarly, a systematic review focusing on robotic surgery for colorectal cancer liver metastases (CRCLM) resection reported a mean 3-year overall survival of 55.25% and a mean 3-year disease-free survival of 37% (111). These findings further support the oncological safety and efficacy of robotic approaches in this context, highlighting their ability to achieve similar long-term results as traditional methods.

The ROBOT4HPB consensus emphasizes the critical need for prospective registries to collect validated outcome metrics for the forthcoming comprehensive assessment of HPB robotics, including crucial long-term oncological data, to provide stronger evidence (76).

General studies comparing robotic surgery outcomes across various cancer types (endometrial, cervical, colorectal, lung, prostate) often show similar long-term outcomes for robotic versus laparoscopic/thoracoscopic and open surgery, without a safety signal requiring further research (119). The increasing utilization of robotic surgery in surgical oncology across various tumor sites, including HPB malignancies, suggests its growing acceptance based on promising short-term outcomes, though continued evaluation of long-term data from large, multicenter, randomized, and prospective studies is crucial for definitive conclusions regarding its role as a standard of care.

Chapter 7: Robotic Liver Surgery in Challenging and Niche Scenarios

The evolution of robotic surgery has profoundly broadened the scope of minimally invasive techniques, extending their applicability to patient populations and anatomical scenarios previously deemed too challenging or complex for traditional laparoscopic approaches. While the pioneering years of robotic liver surgery focused on establishing fundamental feasibility and safety, subsequent advancements have enabled surgeons to confidently tackle increasingly difficult cases. This chapter meticulously explores the role of robotic liver surgery in these demanding situations, including resections for benign liver tumors, transplantations, emergent cases like liver trauma and other abdominal emergencies, and operations in pediatric patients and those with difficult or altered anatomy. The ability of robotic platforms to provide enhanced precision, superior visualization, and improved maneuverability has been instrumental in navigating these intricate scenarios, thereby expanding the benefits of minimally invasive surgery to a wider range of patients within the Hepato-Pancreato-Biliary (HPB) domain.

7.1 Robotic Resection for Benign Liver Tumors

While a significant portion of advanced liver surgical programs appropriately centers on oncological management, the surgical resection of benign liver tumors (BLT) also constitutes a substantial and often complex component of hepatic surgical practice. These lesions, which include diverse pathologies such as large hemangiomas, centrally located adenomas, or focal nodular hyperplasia (FNH), may necessitate surgical intervention due to their size, associated symptoms, potential for complications (e.g., hemorrhage, rupture), or diagnostic uncertainty requiring histological confirmation. Robotic surgery has demonstrably expanded the feasibility and safety of addressing these conditions, particularly as a sophisticated minimally invasive alternative to traditional open or conventional laparoscopic approaches, especially in scenarios presenting inherent challenges (27,64,67).

The categorization of benign liver tumor resection within "Challenging and Niche Scenarios" might initially seem counterintuitive, given the intense focus on malignancy in other chapters. However, the decision to resect benign liver tumors often arises from specific complexities that elevate them beyond routine procedures, making them distinctly challenging and positioning them within a "niche" area of surgical practice.

1. **Anatomical Location and Size**: Benign tumors, despite their non-malignant nature, can often grow to significant sizes or be located in anatomically difficult segments of the liver, such as the caudate lobe or posterior-superior segments. Resection of these deeply located or posterior lesions, especially large ones, presents considerable technical hurdles for minimally invasive approaches due to limited access and maneuverability with conventional laparoscopic instruments. Robotic platforms, with their articulated instruments and enhanced visualization, offer critical advantages in navigating these confined and complex

anatomical spaces, making such resections feasible where they might otherwise require highly invasive open surgery.

2. **Vascularity and Hemorrhage Risk**: Certain benign tumors, notably large hemangiomas or adenomas, can be highly vascular, presenting a substantial risk of intraoperative hemorrhage. Meticulous hemostasis and precise vascular control are paramount during their resection to minimize blood loss and maintain patient stability. The enhanced precision and stable view of robotic systems are particularly beneficial in managing this high vascularity, fitting the theme of tackling technically demanding scenarios.
3. **Preservation of Liver Parenchyma**: For benign conditions, the goal is often to perform parenchyma-sparing resections to preserve as much healthy liver tissue as possible. This requires highly precise dissection and careful delineation of tumor margins, which the robotic platform's enhanced dexterity and 3D visualization facilitate. The ability to

perform such precise anatomical resections in a minimally invasive fashion is a complex refinement.

4. **Diagnostic Uncertainty:** In some cases, benign-appearing lesions may have a small but non-negligible risk of malignancy, necessitating resection for definitive pathological diagnosis. Managing this uncertainty within a minimally invasive framework adds a layer of complexity.

Early systematic reviews of robot-assisted major hepatectomy, which rigorously analyzed initial pioneering cohorts, notably included a significant proportion of benign liver diseases (26.3% of cases), alongside malignant tumors (73.6%). This inclusion in major resection series from the outset underscores that certain benign lesions inherently present a complexity that mandates advanced surgical techniques. These early experiences were instrumental in establishing the safety profile of robotic major resections for non-malignant indications, particularly when dealing with large or deeply situated benign lesions (64). Robotic surgery is indeed being utilized to treat a variety of benign conditions, and studies indicate no deterioration in outcomes when compared to other approaches (27).

When evaluated against open surgery, robotic resection for benign liver diseases has been associated with several quantifiable advantages, including a statistically lower incidence of blood loss, a shorter length of hospital stay, and a reduced overall complication rate. Although studies suggest that peri- and postoperative outcomes for robotic surgery are generally similar to those observed with laparoscopic surgery in this context, robotic platforms offer distinct advantages in overcoming specific technical limitations inherent in conventional laparoscopy. These limitations include constraints imposed by rigid instruments and a two-dimensional (2D) visual field, both of which are particularly restrictive when dealing with large or centrally located benign tumors (67). The enhanced visualization provided by robotic platforms, particularly three-dimensional (3D) high-definition (HD) vision, is crucial for accurately delineating complex benign lesions from healthy liver parenchyma and for meticulous dissection around critical vascular and biliary structures. This improved depth perception and magnification aid significantly in navigating the intricate vascular architecture often encountered with larger or highly vascular benign tumors, such as hemangiomas or large adenomas.

Robotic approaches have consistently demonstrated feasibility and safety for tumors situated in this difficult-to-access segment, including benign lesions, yielding promising postoperative outcomes (68)(69). The ability of robotic systems to provide enhanced precision and maneuverability in such confined and critical anatomical spaces is a direct advantage.

Despite these benefits, the high cost of robotic surgery remains a drawback that can limit its widespread application for benign liver diseases, particularly when clinical benefits do not clearly outweigh costs compared to established laparoscopic methods. More studies are continuously needed to definitively justify the broader introduction of robotic surgery for benign liver diseases and to precisely define the specific patient types that would most optimally benefit from its advanced capabilities (67).

7.2 Robotic Liver Transplantation: Donor, Recipient, and Emerging Scope

Liver transplantation remains one of the most challenging and life-saving operations in abdominal surgery, fundamentally reliant on meticulous dissection and highly precise vascular and biliary anastomoses. The burgeoning field of robotic surgery offers a transformative potential that extends beyond standard resection procedures into this intricate domain. The shift towards minimally invasive techniques in organ transplantation, including the transition from laparoscopic to robotic methods, signifies a notable advancement. Robotic surgery has emerged as a significant development, providing superior precision and outcomes when compared with traditional open approaches in this context (100).

Robotic Living Donor Hepatectomy (LDH): Robotic living donor hepatectomy (LDH), a procedure involving the surgical removal of a portion of a healthy donor's liver for transplantation into a recipient, represents one of the most ethically sensitive, advanced, and technically demanding operations in HPB surgery. The paramount concern in LDH is donor safety, necessitating a minimally invasive approach that minimizes morbidity and ensures rapid recovery. Robotic surgery has emerged as a revolutionary technique in organ transplantation, including liver donation, offering potential benefits that may enhance donor safety and recovery (100). The broader field of organ transplantation is undergoing a revolution significantly influenced by the adoption of minimally invasive techniques, transitioning progressively from laparoscopic to robotic methods. Studies consistently reveal lower morbidity with robotic donor nephrectomy, recipient kidney transplant, and, importantly, robotic donor hepatectomy (100). This accumulating evidence strongly suggests a growing body of support for the benefits of robotic approaches in reducing donor morbidity across various organ procurements, reflecting a positive shift towards less invasive options for living donors. Initial reports, such as the first 12 successful cases of robotic-assisted laparoscopic living donor nephrectomy, demonstrated that the system allows for donor nephrectomy to be performed in a safe and accurate fashion (120).

Robotic liver surgery, including its specific application in living donation, is considered safe and feasible, even if its superiority compared to open and laparoscopic approaches still needs further evaluation. The application of robotic surgery in living donation is still considered to be in its early stages and remains somewhat controversial, with a limited number of published studies (102). Key advantages claimed in favor of robotic surgery for these highly sensitive procedures include three-dimensional (3D) imaging with high definition and a stable view, a more rapid learning curve for surgeons transitioning to this technique compared to laparoscopy, the effective elimination of physiological hand tremors, and significantly enhanced freedom of movement for instruments. These technical benefits are crucial in the precise dissection and meticulous vascular and biliary control required in donor hepatectomy, where minimizing any form of donor morbidity is paramount. Furthermore, most studies comparing robotic to open surgery in this context showed less postoperative pain, less intraoperative blood loss, and a shorter period before the donor returned to normal activity, although operative times may sometimes be longer (102). The excellent outcomes observed can be attributed to the 3D and magnified views, which allow for a better evaluation of the right plane of transection and the complex vascular and biliary anatomy, along with the precision of the robotic movements that facilitate superior bleeding control.

Robotic Liver Transplantation: Recipient and Emerging Scope: While robotic surgery has made substantial inroads into various complex procedures, full robotic recipient liver transplantation (RLT) is not yet widely adopted. This limited adoption is primarily attributed to the extreme complexity of the procedure itself, particularly the critical need for rapid vascular clamping and swift, precise anastomoses during the Anhepatic phase. Despite these challenges, robotic assistance is actively being explored and incrementally applied for specific steps within the recipient liver transplantation procedure.

The current literature suggests that while complete robotic recipient hepatectomy and whole-liver implantation are technically challenging, progress is being made. For instance, initial reports detail the use of robotic assistance for tasks like hilar dissection and preparation of recipient vessels. There is also evidence of robotic techniques being employed for partial hepatectomy in recipient patients, although these remain highly complex and less common procedures. The complexity is compounded by the need to manage various anatomical structures, including the inferior vena cava, hepatic artery, portal vein, and bile duct, often in a tightly confined space.

The potential for robotic assistance in recipient liver transplantation is underscored by its proven capabilities in other demanding procedures. Robotic surgery has demonstrably handled major vascular anastomoses effectively in other fields, such as renal and lung transplantation, and portal vein reconstruction, which are routinely performed with robotic assistance. These established proficiencies suggest a clear pathway for robotic assistance in the recipient hepatectomy phase of liver transplantation, particularly for precise dissection and potentially for complex vascular or biliary anastomoses as technology advances further (94). The inherent advantages of robotic systems, including enhanced dexterity through wristed instruments, superior three-dimensional (3D) visualization, and tremor filtration, provide a level of control and precision that could be highly beneficial for the intricate maneuvers required during recipient hepatectomy and graft implantation (100). Furthermore, the evolution of techniques like robotic donor hepatectomy has paved the way for broader acceptance of robotic methods in transplantation.

A comparative study analyzed the short-term outcomes of fully robotic adult recipient living donor liver transplantation (LDLT) against the traditional open approach. The study included 453 open cases and 54 fully robotic cases. Robotic recipient liver transplantation demonstrated a lower median blood loss (650 ml vs.

2,000 ml, P<0.001), shorter ICU stay (3 vs. 5 days, P<0.001), and shorter hospital stay (14 vs. 20 days, P = 0.030) compared to open surgery. Additionally, the robotic group had fewer infection rates (9.3% vs. 42.8%, P<0.001) and a significantly lower Comprehensive Complication Index® (15.0 vs. 20.9, P=0.045). Regarding survival, the robotic group showed superior recipient survival (100% vs. 91.8%, P=0.040) and comparable 6-month graft survival (98.1% vs. 91.8%, P=0.080). The study concluded that fully robotic recipient LDLT is feasible and safe, offering potential benefits such as reduced morbidity, faster recovery, and shorter hospital stays. These findings support broader adoption of robotic techniques in liver transplantation, though further cost-effectiveness studies and randomized controlled trials are needed (121).

Challenges and Future Directions in Robotic Liver Transplantation: Despite the promising outlook, several significant challenges must be addressed for robotic recipient liver transplantation to become more widespread.

- **Technological Limitations:** Current robotic systems still have limitations that complicate their use in the rapid, time-sensitive environment of recipient hepatectomy. These include the absence of haptic feedback, which is crucial for distinguishing tissue planes and managing fragile vessels, and the need for rapid instrument exchange and re-docking capabilities.
- **Time Sensitivity:** The anhepatic phase of liver transplantation demands extreme speed to minimize cold and warm ischemic time of the donor organ, a factor that current robotic setup and operative times may still challenge.
- **Anesthetic and Physiological Considerations:** Anesthetic considerations for robotic liver transplantation present a unique set of challenges, often related to patient positioning and pneumoperitoneum effects on hemodynamics. These complexities demand a deep understanding of liver disease, liver transplant surgery, and the various implications of robotic surgery to ensure optimal patient outcomes. A

multidisciplinary team approach is critical to manage these intricate physiological responses (101).

- **Learning Curve and Training:** The substantial learning curve associated with these highly complex procedures necessitates structured training programs and significant experience accumulation by the surgical team.

The role of robotics in recipient liver transplantation is still in its early stages and remains an area of active research and development. As robotic technology continues to evolve, incorporating more advanced features like haptic feedback, improved autonomy, and faster setup times, its application in both donor and recipient liver transplantation is expected to further revolutionize treatment paradigms, improve outcomes, and expand the pool of eligible patients. The precision offered by combining medical science, robotics, and engineering is truly revolutionizing surgical specialties. The integration of robotics into liver transplantation and regenerative medicine holds immense promise as a future direction for treating hepatic diseases.

7.3 Robotic Surgery for Liver Trauma and Emergencies

The application of robotic surgery to acute conditions, such as liver trauma and other abdominal emergencies, represents a particularly challenging and evolving frontier in surgical practice. Emergency general surgery (EGS) has traditionally relied heavily on immediate open approaches or, more recently, conventional laparoscopic interventions for acute abdominal pathologies. However, the unique capabilities of robotic platforms are increasingly being explored for their potential benefits in these time-sensitive and high-stakes acute scenarios.

Robotic general surgery, an advanced technology within minimally invasive procedures, is increasingly employed in elective general surgery, showing benefits over laparoscopy in specific cases. While laparoscopy remains a standard approach for common acute abdominal conditions, the role of robotic surgery in emergency general surgery remains uncertain and requires more robust evidence. Early experience with robotics in emergency general surgery suggests that perioperative outcomes can be comparable to laparoscopic surgery in selected conditions, although the associated costs for robotic procedures were notably and significantly higher (28,59). Despite the growing popularity of robotic surgery in the acute care surgical realm, there has been limited research on its utility regarding health outcomes and cost-effectiveness in emergency settings. Current literature indicates some value in utilizing robotic technology in specific urgent procedures, such as cholecystectomies and incarcerated hernia repairs (28). Robotic appendicectomy, for example, is considered safe and feasible, and can be performed in both elective and emergency settings, highlighting its versatility (37).

A review of a single center's experience with emergency robotic surgery demonstrated that it can be a useful and reliable approach, particularly for intraoperative laparoscopic complications, when performed in selected hemodynamically stable patients within very well-trained robotic centers. No conversions to open surgery were reported in this series, and both intraoperative and 30-day mortality rates were 0%, indicating safety in controlled emergent situations (122). These early experiences suggest that the robotic platform might be an effective tool to prevent conversion to open procedures in emergent settings, a significant advantage in acute care where conversion can lead to increased morbidity. Robotic surgery has shown improved perioperative outcomes when compared to an open or laparoscopic approach in these settings (123).

However, concerns continue to exist regarding the widespread adoption of robotic surgery for emergency procedures. These primarily revolve around the immediate availability and accessibility of the robotic platform for emergency units, especially during night shifts, the expected longer operative times associated with setup and docking, and the increased costs compared to conventional approaches. Strict patient selection is consistently advised for emergent general surgery procedures performed with robotics, often limiting its consideration to hemodynamically stable patients who can tolerate the setup time and pneumoperitoneum.

Nevertheless, an emergency setting should not be viewed as an absolute contraindication for robotic surgery if an adequately trained operating surgical team is available and the logistical support is in place. In such conditions, robotic surgery can be considered safe, feasible, and associated with surgical outcomes comparable to a traditional MIS approach. Further research, particularly well-powered large population studies, is needed to definitively determine the true role and widespread applicability of robotic platforms in the emergent setting.

While robot-assisted abdominal aortic surgery has been shown to be technically feasible with acceptable short-term outcomes, it is currently considered only an outlier procedure, with randomized controlled trials being indispensable for its regular use in vascular surgery (124). This highlights the ongoing need for robust evidence even in challenging vascular emergencies that might involve HPB structures. The physiological implications of robotic surgery, such as effects of pneumoperitoneum and steep Trendelenburg positioning on pulmonary compliance and splanchnic perfusion, as well as the potential for reduced surgical stress, are also considerations in emergency cases.

7.4 Robotic Liver Surgery in Pediatric Patients and Difficult Anatomy

The application of robotic liver surgery to pediatric patients and individuals with difficult or altered anatomy represents highly specialized and complex scenarios where the unique technical capabilities of robotic platforms are particularly advantageous.

Robotic Liver Surgery in Pediatric Patients: Pediatric surgery, especially for infants, presents distinct challenges due to their smaller anatomical spaces, more delicate tissues, and specific physiological considerations that differ significantly from adults. Despite these hurdles, minimally invasive surgery (MIS) techniques, including robotic-assisted surgery, are increasingly being applied in pediatric surgery. Robot-assisted pyeloplasty, for example, has become a natural progression from open and laparoscopic procedures in children and is now considered a new gold standard in pediatric minimally invasive surgery. Studies show that robotic pyeloplasty is becoming the preferred procedure for patients with ureteropelvic junction obstruction (UPJO) in children, except for the smallest infants due to limitations in instrument size and the duration of general anesthetic required (125). Robotic pyeloplasty in children is safe and effective with excellent outcomes, even in redo pyeloplasty or challenging anatomical cases, and it can shorten the learning curve for junior surgeons. However, concerns regarding the cost associated with this procedure still exist. The evolution of pediatric robotic surgery continues to lead to advantages for both the patient and surgeon, including shorter postoperative hospital stays, lower pain medication use, and similar success rates relative to open procedures, despite longer operative times (126).

Specific to HPB in pediatrics, robotic surgery for choledochal cysts, which are rare congenital biliary cystic dilations, has shown promising results. Robot-assisted laparoscopic choledochal cystectomy with hepatic-duodenostomy has been associated with overall good outcomes, though anastomotic stenosis is the most common long-term complication. Comparisons of robotic versus laparoscopic surgery for choledochal cyst in children indicate that robotic surgery was associated with significantly lower intraoperative blood loss and shorter postoperative hospital stay, suggesting it is a safe and feasible option for children (127). Robotic-assisted hepaticojejunostomy (RAHJ) in pediatric congenital choledochal dilatation has demonstrated reduced intraoperative bleeding, postoperative complications, and length of stay (128).

The complexity of pediatric liver tumors, which are predominantly primary malignant tumors, demands complete tumor resection with sufficient preservation of liver tissue. The application of 3D visualization technology is crucial for enhancing surgical accuracy in pediatric liver tumors, allowing for precise preoperative planning and intraoperative guidance. Despite the promising results, the utilization of robotic-assisted resections for pediatric tumors has been met with controversy, primarily due to limited data and guidelines regarding patient selection, indications, and long-term oncologic outcomes, which has somewhat delayed its widespread adoption for pediatric tumors (129). The main limitation for robotic pediatric surgery remains the incompatibility between the size of trocars and instruments and the low body weight of children, particularly regarding intercostal space limitations for thoracic procedures (130). Further high-quality prospective observational studies and clinical trials, as well as new technologies specific for the pediatric population, are advisable for robotic procedures to reach the level of the gold standard in pediatric surgery.

Robotic Liver Surgery in Patients with Difficult Anatomy: For patients with difficult anatomy or those with prior abdominal surgeries, robotic liver resection offers notable advantages. These challenges include extensive adhesions from previous operations, distorted anatomical planes, or the complexities associated with managing morbidly obese patients. Prior abdominal surgeries or previous liver resections can lead to extensive and dense adhesions, rendering subsequent operations exceptionally technically challenging and increasing the risk of iatrogenic injury. The robotic platform's articulated instruments and stable 3D visualization can significantly facilitate safe dissection through adhesions and help surgeons navigate altered anatomical planes with enhanced precision. The ability to perform more extensive or complex minimally invasive operations, including repeat resections, is a notable advantage of the robotic approach.

Robotics is also crucial for complex anatomical dissections beyond the liver, providing insights applicable to difficult liver cases. For instance, robotic versus laparoscopic pelvic lateral lymph node dissection showed robotic advantages in harvesting more lymph nodes and fewer complications like urinary retention (131). Similarly, robotic transanal minimally invasive surgery (TAMIS) offers improved ergonomics and versatility in the narrow rectal lumen compared to rigid laparoscopic instruments, suggesting its utility in challenging anatomical fields (132). This technique provides increased dexterity within a small operative field, with the possibility of better surgical precision. In morbidly obese patients, robotic colon surgery has been deemed safe, although high-quality prospective evidence is still needed to confirm specific benefits and oncological safety (133). The precise manipulation and visualization offered by robotics are particularly valuable for achieving quality resections in obese patients with gastric cancer, leading to fewer major complications, despite longer operative times (134). The challenges of implementing new technologies in rural communities also highlight a type of difficult scenario for the adoption of advanced surgical methods. These extensive expansions of robotic capabilities across various complex abdominal and HPB scenarios powerfully underscore its growing and indispensable role in safely managing the most demanding patient cases, extending the benefits of minimally invasive surgery to a broader population, including those with anatomical variations or prior surgical history. The ergonomic superiority of robotic surgery over laparoscopic and open surgery, while still having significant rates of physical strain, contributes to its utility in prolonged and complex cases.

Part IV: Current Status, Training, and Future Directions

Chapter 8: Outcomes, Safety, and Standardization in Robotic Liver Surgery

The advent of robotic platforms has profoundly reshaped the landscape of liver surgery, building upon the foundational shifts initiated by minimally invasive techniques. This chapter meticulously examines the current status of robotic liver surgery, focusing on its comparative outcomes against established laparoscopic and open approaches, its safety profile, and strategies for complication management, the analysis of key intraoperative parameters, and the critical efforts towards standardization of techniques and reporting. The progression of surgical robotics from its early conceptualization in general surgery to its specialized application in hepatobiliary (HPB) procedures underscores a continuous quest for enhanced precision and reduced invasiveness.

8.1 Comparative Outcomes: Robotic vs. Laparoscopic vs. Open Approaches

The evolution of surgical techniques for liver resection has seen a progressive shift from traditional open approaches to minimally invasive methods, initially through laparoscopy and more recently, with the integration of robotic platforms. Comparative studies are essential to delineate the advantages and disadvantages of each modality, providing an evidence-based foundation for their respective roles in modern hepatic surgery.

Robotic vs. Laparoscopic Liver Resection: Robotic liver resection (RLR) has emerged as a significant advancement, designed to overcome several inherent technical limitations of conventional laparoscopic liver resection. The primary advantages offered by robotic systems include enhanced dexterity through articulated instruments ("endo-wrists"), a stable, high-resolution three-dimensional (3D) magnified field of view, and tremor-filtering technology, which collectively contribute to increased surgical precision.

Multiple studies and meta-analyses have compared the perioperative and oncological outcomes of RLR and LLR, particularly for complex resections.

- **Feasibility and Safety:** Both RLR and LLR are considered feasible and safe for selected patients (8,54). However, the robotic platform's technical advantages may allow for the safe performance of more complex or extended resections that would be challenging or deemed impossible laparoscopically (8,31)
- **Intraoperative Blood Loss**: RLR is frequently associated with less estimated intraoperative blood loss compared to LLR (22,69). For instance, a meta-analysis on difficult posterosuperior segments showed RLR had less estimated blood loss and fewer blood transfusions than LLR (69).
- **Operative Time:** Operative times for RLR can vary. Some studies report longer operative times for RLR, especially during the early phases of adoption, due to setup and docking (31,34). However, other studies, particularly for complex resections like those in posterosuperior segments, suggest shorter operative times with RLR (69).

- **Conversion to Open Surgery**: RLR may offer a lower rate of conversion to open surgery compared to LLR, particularly for challenging cases or those in anatomically difficult locations (69,78). This is attributed to the superior control and maneuverability provided by the robotic system.
- **Postoperative Complications and Morbidity**: Overall postoperative morbidity rates are generally comparable between RLR and LLR (54,69).
- **Length of Hospital Stay**: Both minimally invasive approaches offer shorter hospital stays compared to open surgery. Between RLR and LLR, the length of hospital stay is often comparable or slightly shorter for RLR (22,31).
- **Oncological Outcomes:** For malignant lesions such as hepatocellular carcinoma (HCC) and colorectal liver metastases (CRLM), RLR has demonstrated oncological outcomes equivalent to LLR, including R0 resection rates and long-term survival (31,66). This suggests that the

technical advantages of robotics do not compromise oncological radicality.

Robotic vs. Open Liver Resection: The comparison of robotic liver resection with traditional open liver resection (OLR) typically highlights the well-established benefits of minimally invasive surgery.

- **Reduced Invasiveness Benefits**: RLR, similar to LLR, offers the benefits of minimally invasive surgery, including smaller incisions, reduced postoperative pain, lower blood loss, fewer wound complications, and quicker patient recovery (8,22)
- **Blood Loss and Transfusion Rates:** RLR is consistently associated with significantly less intraoperative blood loss and lower rates of blood transfusion compared to OLR (22).
- **Length of Hospital Stay**: Patients undergoing RLR generally experience a shorter length of hospital stay than

those undergoing OLR, facilitating faster return to normal activities (22,31).

- **Morbidity and Mortality:** While overall mortality rates are low across all approaches for selected patients, RLR often shows comparable or even reduced overall morbidity compared to OLR, especially for complex cases (8,22).
- **Oncological Equivalence:** For liver malignancies, robotic hepatectomy has demonstrated oncological outcomes (e.g., R0 resection rates, lymph node yield, long-term survival) that are equivalent to open approaches for appropriately selected patients (22,31).

Overall Comparative Landscape: While there is a growing consensus on the safety and feasibility of RLR, particularly for anterior and left lateral sectionectomies, and increasingly for posterosuperior or major resections, the definitive superiority of RLR over LLR in all contexts is still a subject of ongoing debate and research. Many studies show non-inferiority rather than clear superiority, especially for less complex resections. The choice of approach often depends on tumor location, complexity, surgeon experience, and institutional resources. However, for specific technically demanding resections, such as those in the posterior-superior segments or caudate lobe, the robotic platform's inherent advantages often make it the preferred minimally invasive modality (68,69). The increased cost associated with robotic systems remains a notable factor to consider in this comparative analysis.

8.2 Safety Profile and Complication Management

The safety profile of robotic liver surgery (RLS) is a critical aspect of its adoption and widespread integration into clinical practice, particularly given the inherent complexity and high stakes of hepatic resections. While advancements in robotic technology aim to enhance precision and control, a thorough understanding of potential complications and their effective management is paramount to ensuring optimal patient outcomes.

Overall Safety and Feasibility: Numerous studies and systematic reviews consistently affirm the feasibility and safety of RLS for a broad range of indications, from minor to major hepatectomies (8,54). The distinct advantages of robotic systems, such as high-definition three-dimensional (3D) visualization, articulated instruments (endo-wrists) providing seven degrees of freedom, and tremor filtration, contribute to improved dexterity and precision. These technological benefits are particularly valuable in the highly vascular and anatomically intricate hepatic milieu, helping surgeons navigate complex structures and perform delicate dissections with enhanced control.

Common and Major Complications: While RLS generally demonstrates a safety profile comparable to, or in some aspects superior to, traditional laparoscopic and open approaches, specific complications remain a focus of vigilance and management.

- **Intraoperative Hemorrhage:** Despite the robotic system's ability to provide precise hemostasis and reduce overall blood loss, significant intraoperative bleeding can still occur, particularly in major resections or complex tumor cases.

However, studies often show a decreased or at least equivalent amount of intraoperative blood loss with RLS compared to conventional techniques (22,69). The 3D view and fine instrument control aid in the early identification and management of bleeding sources.

- **Bile Leak:** Bile leakage is a recognized complication following liver resection, regardless of the approach. The meticulous dissection facilitated by robotic systems and enhanced visualization, including the use of indocyanine green (ICG) fluorescence imaging for real-time bile duct mapping, can aid in reducing the incidence or severity of bile leaks (25,83). Nevertheless, careful identification and ligation of small biliary radicals remain critical.
- **Postoperative Liver Failure (POLF):** This severe complication is largely dependent on the patient's underlying liver function and the volume/quality of the remnant liver, rather than solely on the surgical approach. However, the precision of RLS and its potential for less tissue

manipulation may theoretically contribute to preserving hepatic function. Careful patient selection and preoperative assessment of liver function are crucial in mitigating this risk (66).

- **Infections and Wound Complications:** As a minimally invasive procedure, RLS typically results in smaller incisions, which inherently reduces the risk of wound-related complications such as infection and dehiscence compared to open surgery. Postoperative infection rates are generally low, consistent with other minimally invasive procedures.
- **Conversion to Open Surgery:** Conversion to open surgery is a measure of the technical difficulty encountered during a minimally invasive procedure and an important safety outcome. While the aim is to complete the procedure minimally invasively, conversion is considered a safe alternative when unexpected complexities arise. Robotic platforms, due to their enhanced capabilities, may offer a lower conversion rate compared to conventional

laparoscopy, particularly for difficult resections (69)(122).

Risk Factors and Patient Selection: Careful patient selection is paramount for ensuring the safety and success of RLS. Factors considered include the patient's overall health, comorbidities, tumor characteristics (size, location, proximity to major vascular structures), and the presence of underlying liver disease (e.g., cirrhosis). For patients with cirrhosis, RLS may offer advantages due to minimized trauma to fragile liver parenchyma, which can help preserve remnant liver function and mitigate the risk of complications from portal hypertension. Similarly, for patients requiring repeat resections with extensive adhesions, the robotic system's maneuverability can facilitate safer dissection (22,31).

Complication Management and Intraoperative Monitoring: Effective complication management in RLS relies on a combination of advanced intraoperative techniques and robust postoperative protocols.

- **Enhanced Visualization and Intraoperative Imaging:**

The 3D magnified view provided by robotic systems allows for superior identification of anatomical structures and potential areas of bleeding or bile leakage. The integration of advanced imaging modalities such as ICG fluorescence imaging provides real-time anatomical and functional guidance, crucial for identifying liver segments, vascular structures, and biliary anatomy, thereby enhancing safety and accuracy. Intraoperative ultrasound (IOUS) integrated with robotic platforms further aids in tumor localization, margin assessment, and visualization of deep vascular structures, particularly when haptic feedback is absent.

- **Precision and Stability:** The tremor-filtering and motion-scaling capabilities of robotic systems allow for extremely fine and stable dissection, reducing the risk of iatrogenic injury to critical vascular and biliary structures. This precision is invaluable for achieving meticulous hemostasis and preventing inadvertent damage during parenchymal transection.

- **Multidisciplinary Team Approach:** Successful management of complications and optimized patient outcomes in complex HPB surgery, including RLS, depends heavily on a well-coordinated multidisciplinary team. This includes skilled anesthesiologists, intensivists, nurses, and surgical assistants who are familiar with robotic procedures and potential challenges. The surgeon, while at the console, relies on effective communication and teamwork from the bedside assistant.
- **Perioperative Protocols:** Adherence to enhanced recovery after surgery (ERAS) protocols and standardized complication management pathways helps to optimize patient recovery and mitigate adverse events. These protocols are designed to minimize surgical stress, manage pain effectively, and facilitate early mobilization and nutritional intake, contributing to overall safety and reducing hospital stay.

Learning Curve and Experience: While RLS offers significant advantages, overcoming the learning curve is crucial for maintaining a high safety profile. Studies emphasize that complex robotic liver resections are considered safe and feasible once the surgical team has plateaued on their learning curve (8). Experienced surgeons and high-volume centers consistently report better outcomes, underscoring the importance of structured training and mentorship (66). Standardized education and certification programs are deemed critical for future generations of surgeons to ensure patient safety as robotic surgery expands (33).

8.3 Intraoperative Parameters: Blood Loss and Hospital Stay

The assessment of intraoperative parameters, particularly estimated blood loss (EBL) and operative time, along with postoperative metrics such as length of hospital stay (LOS), provides crucial insights into the efficiency, safety, and patient benefits of different surgical approaches in liver surgery. Robotic liver surgery (RLS) has demonstrated notable advantages in these areas when compared to traditional methods, stemming from its advanced technical features (8,22)

Blood Loss and Transfusion Rates: One of the most consistently reported benefits of minimally invasive liver surgery, including RLS, is the reduction in intraoperative blood loss. The highly vascular nature of the liver parenchyma makes meticulous hemostasis paramount during resection. Robotic systems, with their enhanced capabilities, contribute significantly to this reduction (22).

- The high-definition, three-dimensional (3D) magnified visualization provides an immersive view of the surgical field, allowing for precise identification of even small vessels and accurate delineation of resection planes. This improved depth perception enables surgeons to perform finer dissections and achieve more selective vascular control.

- Articulated instruments, known as "endo-wrists," mimic the human hand's seven degrees of freedom, enabling unparalleled dexterity and articulation within confined spaces. This allows for meticulous dissection, precise control of vessels, and the ability to perform complex intracorporeal suturing with greater ease and accuracy, which are critical for effective hemostasis.
- Tremor-filtering technology and motion scaling functions translate larger, less precise hand movements from the surgeon's console into smaller, more stable instrument movements within the patient, thereby minimizing inadvertent tissue trauma and promoting controlled dissection. This stability is particularly advantageous when working around major vascular structures.

Studies comparing RLS to conventional laparoscopic liver resection (LLR) and open liver resection (OLR) frequently report lower EBL in the robotic group. For example, RLS has been consistently associated with a decreased or at least equal amount of intraoperative blood loss compared to both conventional laparoscopic and open techniques (22). A meta-analysis focusing on robotic versus laparoscopic liver resection for challenging posterosuperior segments showed that RLS was associated with less estimated blood loss and fewer blood transfusions. Reduced blood loss directly correlates with lower transfusion rates, minimizing the associated risks and costs of blood products (69).

Operative Time: Operative time in robotic surgery is a multifactorial parameter influenced by procedure complexity, surgeon experience (learning curve), and the specific steps involved in setting up the robotic platform.

- Initial phases of robotic adoption, and for less common or more complex procedures, may involve longer operative times due to the time required for robot docking, instrument exchanges, and the surgical team's adaptation to the new workflow (31,34).

- However, as surgeons progress beyond the initial learning curve, operative times tend to decrease and can become comparable to, or even shorter than, those of laparoscopic approaches for certain complex procedures. For instance, the meta-analysis on difficult posterosuperior segments noted shorter operative times with RLS compared to LLR (69).
- The ergonomic benefits, reduced fatigue, and enhanced precision offered by the robotic system can potentially contribute to maintaining efficiency during prolonged and intricate liver resections (1,10).

Length of Hospital Stay (LOS): Minimally invasive approaches, including RLS, have consistently demonstrated a significant advantage in reducing the length of hospital stay compared to open liver surgery. This reduction in LOS is a key benefit for patients and healthcare systems, leading to faster recovery and reduced healthcare costs.

- The less invasive nature of RLS results in smaller incisions, leading to less postoperative pain, reduced need for opioid analgesics, and a quicker return of bowel function. These factors contribute directly to faster patient mobilization and earlier discharge.
- Studies comparing RLS to LLR often show comparable, or sometimes even shorter, hospital stays for robotic procedures. Robotic hepatectomy can provide patients with more rapid recovery and a shorter hospital stay, which can help offset the substantial costs of robot acquisition and maintenance (31).
- The cumulative benefits of reduced blood loss, lower complication rates, and optimized perioperative care (including Enhanced Recovery After Surgery protocols (82))contribute to this expedited recovery and shorter inpatient stay, improving overall patient satisfaction and resource utilization.

Overall, the data on intraoperative parameters and hospital stay consistently highlight the benefits of robotic liver surgery in terms of reduced blood loss and shorter hospitalizations, reinforcing its role as a valuable minimally invasive technique in selected patients and complex scenarios.

8.4 Standardization of Techniques and Reporting

The rapid evolution and increasing adoption of robotic liver surgery (RLS) necessitate robust efforts towards standardization of surgical techniques, training, and outcome reporting. Standardization is crucial for several reasons: it ensures patient safety, facilitates effective training and skill acquisition, allows for meaningful comparison of outcomes across different institutions and studies, and ultimately promotes the safe and widespread integration of this advanced technology into mainstream practice.

Importance of Standardization: In a burgeoning field like RLS, which builds upon the foundations of conventional minimally invasive surgery, heterogeneity in surgical approaches, patient selection criteria, and outcome assessment can obscure clear evidence of efficacy and safety. Standardization aims to mitigate these challenges by:

- **Enhancing Patient Safety:** By defining best practices and establishing consistent protocols, standardization helps minimize variability in care, thereby reducing the risk of complications and ensuring predictable outcomes (33). Safety protocols, including those for emergent conversion to open surgery, must be diligently put in place and reviewed before every procedure to ensure safety (32).
- **Facilitating Training and Skill Acquisition:** A structured and standardized curriculum for robotic surgical training is essential for young surgeons to achieve proficiency and adapt to a wide range of surgical applications. The learning curve for various robotic procedures is recognized, and formal training pathways, often incorporating simulation and virtual reality, are crucial to overcome it safely (4,45–47,50,135).

- **Enabling Comparative Analysis and Evidence Generation:** Consistent reporting of data is fundamental for conducting high-quality research, such as larger, well-designed prospective studies and randomized trials, which are needed to definitively analyze the true value and long-term impact of robotic surgery. Early retrospective case studies were often difficult to compare due to methodological variations and limited sample sizes (8,29).

Key Areas for Standardization:

1. **Standardization of Surgical Techniques:** The anatomical complexity of the liver necessitates precise surgical techniques. Standardization involves defining clear steps and approaches for different types of robotic liver resections, from minor segmentectomies to complex major hepatectomies. This includes techniques for parenchymal transection, vascular control, and biliary management (25).

For instance, systematic extrahepatic Glissonean pedicle isolation, an anatomical technique considered essential for safe and curable liver resection, can be standardized by a comprehensive understanding of liver anatomy based on structures like Laennec's capsule. This approach aims to minimize parenchymal destruction and improve surgical precision (65).

2. **Standardization of Training and Education:** Achieving proficiency in RLS requires specific and extensive training in both hepato-biliary surgery and broader minimally invasive surgical techniques. Standardized education and certification programs are crucial for ensuring patient safety for future generations of surgeons considering robotic surgery. These programs often utilize commercial virtual reality simulators as a primary component of their training, instrumental in aiding surgeons to learn basic robotics skills and practice procedural activities in a safe and controlled environment. Mentorship by experienced robotic surgeons

also plays a vital role. Establishing credentialing and competency maintenance pathways ensures ongoing skill proficiency.

3. **Standardization of Reporting and Outcome Metrics:** To accurately assess the efficacy and safety of RLS, consistent and standardized reporting of outcomes is indispensable. This includes:
   - **Perioperative Outcomes:** Standardized reporting of intraoperative parameters such as estimated blood loss, operative time, and conversion rates.
   - **Postoperative Morbidity and Mortality:** Consistent use of validated classification systems, such as the Clavien-Dindo classification, to grade postoperative complications ensures uniform data collection and comparison across studies. Overall morbidity and mortality rates are key safety indicators.
   - **Length of Hospital Stay:** Standardized reporting of

LOS facilitates comparison of recovery trajectories and resource utilization.

- **Oncological Outcomes:** For malignant diseases, standardized reporting of R0 resection rates (negative margins), lymph node yield, recurrence rates, disease-free survival (DFS), and overall survival (OS) is critical to establish oncological equivalence or superiority. The comparability of currently available retrospective case studies for complex procedures, like robotic liver resections, is often difficult due to variations in methodologies and limited sample sizes, underscoring the need for more rigorous data.

4. **Standardization of Patient Selection Criteria:** Defining clear and consistent criteria for patient selection is fundamental to achieving optimal outcomes and avoiding unsuitable cases for robotic intervention. This involves considering factors such as tumor size and location, patient

comorbidities, and the presence of underlying liver disease, particularly cirrhosis. Standardized guidelines ensure that the benefits of RLS are extended to appropriately selected patients while mitigating risks in complex scenarios.

Consensus Guidelines and Registries: Recognizing the imperative for standardization, international expert groups and professional societies have begun to develop consensus guidelines for robotic HPB surgery. The ROBOT4HPB conference, for instance, initiated a multidisciplinary effort to establish the first guidelines on the safety and indications of robotics in HPB surgery, including liver procedures. These guidelines emphasize the importance of expertise and the need for prospective registries to collect validated outcome metrics for comprehensive assessment of HPB robotics, thereby providing stronger evidence for its widespread adoption and defining priorities for future research. Such registries are vital for systematically capturing long-term oncological data and other patient-important outcomes to inform ongoing practice. The increasing utilization of robotic surgery demands continuous evaluation through rigorous research to ensure its sustained growth and benefit to patients (30,76).

Ahmad Mahamid

Chapter 9: Training, Education, and Simulation in Robotic Liver Surgery

The transformative impact of robotic surgical systems on the landscape of liver surgery, while offering unparalleled precision and dexterity, concurrently introduces a critical demand for robust and standardized training and education. The successful integration of these advanced platforms, particularly in complex hepatobiliary (HPB) procedures, hinges not only on technological sophistication but profoundly on the proficiency and competence of the surgical team. This chapter delves into the multifaceted aspects of establishing effective robotic liver surgery programs, the indispensable role of simulation and mentorship in skill acquisition, and the crucial frameworks for credentialing and competency maintenance, all within the historical and evolutionary context that has paved the way for modern HPB applications.

9.1 Establishing Robotic Liver Surgery Programs and Structured Training

The successful implementation of robotic surgery programs across various institutions necessitates a comprehensive, multidisciplinary team approach, demanding significant commitment and investment from clinical faculty, operating room staff, and hospital administrators. This institutional commitment is foundational for creating an environment conducive to learning and safe practice.

Foundational Requirements for Program Establishment: Establishing a new robotic liver surgery program or expanding an existing one requires careful planning and resource allocation. Key elements include:

- **Infrastructure Investment:** This encompasses the acquisition of robotic platforms, ensuring adequate space in operating rooms, and the necessary supporting equipment. The substantial financial costs involved in both acquiring and subsequently maintaining these advanced robotic systems constitute a primary and pervasive concern that institutions must address.

- **Team Development:** The entire surgical team, not just the operating surgeon, requires specialized training. This includes anesthesiologists, intensivists, nurses, and surgical assistants, whose expertise and commitment to patient care are invaluable for successful outcomes in robotic procedures. Workflow and teamwork can be impacted in robot-assisted surgery due to the surgeon being physically positioned away from the patient's bedside, highlighting the need for effective communication and coordination.
- **Strategic Planning:** The growth of robot-assisted surgery in the liver has unfolded as a deliberate stepwise approach, unlike the rapid adoption seen in simpler procedures like laparoscopic cholecystectomy. This controlled growth allows for the identification of critical areas for improvement, many of which reside at the intricate nexus of advanced engineering and precise medical practice.

Structured Training Pathways: A recognized learning curve is inherently associated with various robotic procedures, meaning a period of dedicated practice and training is required for surgeons to achieve proficiency. To facilitate this, robotic surgical training requires systematization for young surgeons, aiming to standardize it and enable adaptation to a wider range of surgical applications.

- **Curriculum Development:** Structured training pathways have been developed to guide surgeons through the skill acquisition process. These curricula typically encompass both preclinical phases (e.g., didactic lectures, simulator practice) and subsequent clinical phases, with the latter specifically focusing on the practical introduction of the robotic platform into surgical practice under supervision. The European Hernia Society, for example, describes a training curriculum for robot-assisted abdominal wall surgery that is contingent upon the specific robot platform, the surgeon's prior experience in other abdominal procedures, and their existing expertise in abdominal wall repair techniques (48). While this example is from hernia surgery, the principle of structured, experience-contingent training is universally applicable across robotic specialties, including liver surgery.

- **Phased Implementation:** For complex procedures such as robotic liver resections, a phased approach to training is often advocated, progressing from simpler cases (e.g., peripheral resections) to more complex ones (e.g., major hepatectomies, centrally located tumors) as proficiency is gained. Achieving consistently excellent clinical outcomes and ensuring optimal patient safety in HPB robotic procedures necessitates specific and extensive training in both highly specialized hepato-biliary surgery and broader general minimally invasive surgical techniques to effectively overcome this learning curve.
- **Learning Curve Considerations:** Studies have indicated that the learning curve for specific robotic procedures, such as robotic right colectomy, can be significantly faster when

> compared to laparoscopic approaches (49). This suggests that the ergonomic and technical advantages of robotics may accelerate the acquisition of certain skills. However, the overall complexity of liver surgery means that while the robotic *platform* may offer a shortened learning curve for surgeons when compared to laparoscopic approaches for extensive operations (31), a substantial training period is still required for the complex decision-making and critical maneuvers unique to hepatic procedures.

Ensuring patient safety through standardized education and certification for the future generation of surgeons, considering robotic surgery is a critical measure as the use of robots in surgery continues to expand.

9.2 The Role of Simulation and Mentorship

The inherent complexity and recognized learning curve associated with robotic liver surgery (RLS) underscore the critical roles of simulation and mentorship in fostering surgeon proficiency and ensuring patient safety. These educational modalities provide controlled environments for skill acquisition and pathways for knowledge transfer from experienced practitioners to those new to the robotic platform.

The Role of Simulation: Simulation plays a crucial and increasingly prominent role in skill acquisition for robotic surgery. It allows surgeons to practice and refine technical skills in a risk-free environment before applying them to live patients.

- **Types of Simulation:** Robotic surgery curricula extensively utilize commercial virtual reality (VR) simulators as a primary component of their training programs. These advanced simulators are instrumental in aiding surgeons to learn basic robotics skills and to practice procedural activities effectively (50,135). Beyond VR, other simulation modalities include dry lab and wet lab training, as well as cadaveric models, which offer varying degrees of realism and tactile feedback (23).

- **Benefits of Simulation:**
    - **Safe Learning Environment:** Simulation provides a platform where errors can occur without patient harm, allowing for iterative practice and immediate feedback. This is particularly important given the high stakes of liver surgery.
    - **Objective Performance Assessment:** Many simulators offer objective performance metrics (OPMs) that measure instrument movements and surgical technical skills (136). These objective measures provide quantitative feedback for training and skill acquisition, helping surgeons identify areas for improvement and track progress.
    - **Accelerated Skill Acquisition:** Deliberate practice on simulators has been shown to accelerate the learning curve for robotic procedures. The ability to repeatedly perform specific tasks, such as intracorporeal suturing or precise dissection, builds

muscle memory and enhances dexterity (50).

  - **Skill Transferability:** Skills acquired in a simulated environment can be transferred to the operating room, improving actual surgical performance. This is critical for procedures requiring complex maneuvers, such as those within the confined anatomical spaces of the abdomen.

- **Integration into Training Programs:** Simulation is widely integrated into structured robotic surgical training pathways. This often involves a stepwise progression from basic skills modules to more complex procedural simulations, culminating in a demonstrable level of proficiency before clinical application (50). Video-based educational tools in robotic surgery have also demonstrably shown a positive effect on educational outcomes, proving particularly valuable for skill development when used as a review tool (51).

The Role of Mentorship: Mentorship, particularly from experienced robotic surgeons, is an indispensable component of training in complex surgical fields like RLS. While simulation builds foundational technical skills, mentorship provides the nuanced guidance necessary for clinical judgment, strategic decision-making, and navigating the complexities of actual patient cases (45,66).

- **Expert Contributions:** Expert contributions from pioneering surgeons and the establishment of high-volume centers have been instrumental in meticulously defining and refining robotic surgical techniques and consistently demonstrating the fundamental feasibility and safety of these advanced procedures (25).
- **Types of Mentorships:**
  - **Direct Supervision:** Initially, trainees perform procedures under the direct, hands-on supervision of a qualified robotic surgeon. This allows for real-time guidance and intervention.

- **Dual-Console Training:** The da Vinci system's dual-console capability allows a mentor to observe, guide, and even intervene directly from a second console, facilitating interactive training and immediate feedback during live cases. This is particularly valuable for teaching intricate maneuvers and problem-solving in real-time (4).
- **Telementoring:** The concept of Telementoring, where an expert guides a remote surgeon via telecommunication, is an emerging aspect that could expand access to specialized mentorship, particularly in areas with limited robotic expertise. This aligns with the broader application of robotics for remote operation (2).

- **Benefits of Mentorship:** Mentors guide trainees through the nuances of patient selection, intraoperative decision-making, and complication management. They impart not only technical skills but also critical non-technical skills such as communication, teamwork, and leadership, which are vital for successful outcomes in robot-assisted surgery where the surgeon is physically positioned away from the patient's bedside. The transferability of skills and experience across the HPB domain is evident in pancreatic surgery, where early reports showed encouraging results with morbidity and mortality comparable to open surgery, indicating the value of experienced mentors (63).

- **Overcoming the Learning Curve:** For complex procedures like robotic pancreaticoduodenectomy, participating surgeons who had already surpassed their individual learning curves showed safe and feasible outcomes, underscoring the importance of mentorship in reaching proficiency (75). The advantages of a robotic approach to liver resection specifically include a shortened learning curve for surgeons when compared to laparoscopic approaches, facilitating a quicker path to proficiency under proper guidance (31).

The combined approach of structured simulation training and expert mentorship is fundamental to developing competent robotic liver surgeons, enabling them to navigate the complexities of hepatic anatomy and pathology with precision and safety.

9.3 Credentialing and Competency Maintenance

As robotic liver surgery (RLS) continues to integrate into mainstream clinical practice, the establishment of robust credentialing processes and ongoing competency maintenance frameworks becomes paramount. These measures are essential to ensure patient safety, uphold surgical quality, and maintain public trust in this technologically advanced field. The inherent complexity of hepatic procedures, coupled with the unique demands of the robotic platform, necessitates a structured approach to validate and sustain surgeon proficiency.

Credentialing for Robotic Liver Surgery: Credentialing refers to the process by which healthcare organizations formally grant permission for a practitioner to provide specific services, based on their qualifications and demonstrated competence. For robotic surgery, this often involves a multi-faceted evaluation:

- **Prerequisite Surgical Experience:** Candidates typically must possess a strong foundation in general surgery and, more specifically, in minimally invasive hepatobiliary surgery. This ensures that they have the fundamental anatomical knowledge and surgical judgment necessary before learning the robotic interface (66).
- **Structured Training Completion:** Completion of a standardized training curriculum is a core requirement. This usually includes didactic learning, extensive simulator practice (both basic skills and procedure-specific modules), and potentially inanimate or animate laboratory experience. Many robotic surgery curricula extensively utilize commercial virtual reality simulators as a primary component of their training programs (50,135).
- **Proctored Cases:** A critical component of initial credentialing involves performing a specified number of

robotic cases under the direct supervision of an experienced robotic surgeon. This proctoring ensures that the trainee can safely and effectively apply their learned skills in a live clinical setting. The specific number of proctored cases required can vary by institution or professional society guidelines (66).

- **Assessment of Proficiency:** Beyond simply completing training modules, a demonstration of proficiency is required. This can include passing a standardized objective assessment on simulators or a formal evaluation of operative videos by expert reviewers (136). The European Hernia Society, for instance, describes a training curriculum for robot-assisted abdominal wall surgery that is contingent upon the surgeon's prior experience and existing expertise, highlighting the importance of tailored assessment (48).

Competency Maintenance: Given the continuous evolution of robotic platforms, instrumentation, and surgical techniques, initial credentialing alone is insufficient to guarantee lifelong proficiency.

Ongoing competency maintenance is crucial, ensuring surgeons remain up-to-date and maintain their skill levels.

- **Continuing Medical Education (CME):** Participation in advanced robotic surgery courses, workshops, and scientific conferences helps surgeons stay abreast of new developments and refine their techniques.
- **Case Volume and Outcomes Monitoring:** Regular review of case logs and outcomes data, including intraoperative parameters, complication rates, and oncological results (if applicable), is vital. High-volume centers often demonstrate better outcomes, underscoring the importance of sustained practice.
- **Re-certification or Re-privileging:** Institutions or professional bodies may require periodic re-evaluation of robotic surgical skills, potentially through simulator-based assessments, video reviews, or renewed proctoring. Objective performance metrics (OPMs) derived from instrument movements and surgical technical skills are being

developed to assess and improve surgeon performance, providing objective feedback for skill maintenance.

- **Peer Review and Quality Assurance:** Engagement in peer review processes and institutional quality assurance programs helps identify areas for improvement and ensures adherence to best practices (32).

Challenges and Future Directions: Despite the recognized importance, challenges remain in standardizing credentialing and competency maintenance across institutions and countries. Variability in training standards and a lack of universal guidelines can lead to inconsistencies. The significant cost associated with simulation technology and the time commitment for ongoing training also present barriers.

Future directions for competency maintenance in robotic liver surgery include further integration of artificial intelligence (AI) and advanced analytics into training and assessment (137). AI in robot-assisted surgery is exploring efficacy in improving patient safety through applications like motion analysis, training, and tissue retraction. Automated performance metrics, supported by AI, could provide more frequent and objective assessments of surgical skills, potentially revolutionizing how competency is tracked and maintained over a surgeon's career (136). The establishment of consensus guidelines, such as those formulated by the ROBOT4HPB conference, represents a collaborative and multidisciplinary initiative to provide standardized recommendations on training, expertise, and outcome assessment in HPB robotics, thereby promoting safer and more effective practice (76).

Ahmad Mahamid

Chapter 10: The Future of Robotic Liver Surgery: Innovations and Uncharted Territories

The trajectory of robotic surgery, a journey marked by continuous and groundbreaking innovation, has relentlessly pushed the boundaries of minimally invasive techniques from their pioneering scopes towards an era defined by unprecedented precision healing. Within the profoundly intricate domain of hepatobiliary (HPB) surgery, this technological evolution has been particularly impactful, directly addressing the complex anatomical and physiological challenges inherently associated with liver interventions. As we gaze forward, the future landscape of robotic liver surgery is poised for nothing less than a profound and transformative revolution, a revolution driven by the synergistic advancements in artificial intelligence (AI), increasingly sophisticated image-guided technologies, and entirely novel, next-generation robotic platforms. These forthcoming innovations promise to further augment human surgical capabilities, dramatically enhance patient safety, and fundamentally expand the operative spectrum into realms previously deemed unattainable by conventional means. The integration of these cutting-edge, yet-to-be-fully-realized technologies reflects an unyielding and relentless pursuit of superior patient outcomes, aiming to redefine surgical precision, significantly improve operational efficiency, and comprehensively overcome existing limitations in the surgical management of complex liver pathologies. This chapter will strictly focus on truly future, emerging, and speculative technologies, including advanced AI, Augmented Reality (AR), Virtual Reality (VR), and next-generation robotic platforms that are primarily in the research, early clinical trial, or conceptual phase, projecting their transformative future impact on liver surgery.

10.1 Artificial Intelligence and Image-Guided Surgery

The confluence of Artificial Intelligence (AI) and advanced image-guided surgery (IGS) represents a pivotal and transformative frontier in the ongoing evolution of robotic liver surgery, promising to usher in an era of unparalleled precision, sophisticated predictive capabilities, and highly standardized care. These revolutionary technologies aim to fundamentally transcend current surgical limitations by providing real-time, highly granular, and data-driven insights, coupled with profoundly augmented intraoperative guidance (138).

Artificial Intelligence in Future Robotic Surgery: Artificial intelligence, encompassing the powerful methodologies of machine learning and deep learning, is increasingly being conceptualized and applied to future robotic surgery with the overarching goal of standardizing complex techniques, dramatically increasing surgical efficiency, and ultimately reducing clinical complications. The seamless integration of advanced AI algorithms into future robotic platforms promises to profoundly enhance surgical performance by providing intelligent assistance and sophisticated decision support for complex surgical endeavors (138,139).

- **Surgical Performance Optimization and Learning:** Future AI systems will possess the capability to meticulously analyze vast and diverse amounts of surgical data, including intricate video feeds and precise instrument movements, to identify optimal surgical steps, predict potential intraoperative challenges, and ultimately forecast patient outcomes. This data-driven paradigm will facilitate the development of advanced automated performance metrics (APMs) that objectively and quantitatively measure instrument movements and refined surgical technical skills, designed to assess and significantly improve surgeon performance. These objective measures will provide granular quantitative feedback for future training and skill acquisition, thereby contributing to a more standardized and data-informed approach to surgical excellence by precisely quantifying proficiency. Such advanced AI analysis will also lead to the dynamic generation of "surgical atlases" or "roadmaps" that meticulously delineate optimal trajectories and critical maneuvers for specific future surgical procedures, providing an unprecedented level of guidance (136,138).

- **Intraoperative Decision Support and Predictive Analytics:** Future AI algorithms will possess the capacity to process complex intraoperative imaging data and real-time physiological metrics, enabling them to offer highly sophisticated, real-time recommendations that could intelligently guide surgeons through complex anatomical variations or challenging dissection planes. This capability will extend into truly predictive analytics, where advanced AI models can forecast the likelihood of future postoperative outcomes, such as the risk of postoperative liver failure (POLF) or tumor recurrence, based on comprehensive preoperative patient characteristics, real-time intraoperative events, and the planned resection volume. While it was noted that conclusive proof regarding currently available AI systems reliably identifying critical tasks determining patient outcomes was limited in early stages, active research is vigorously exploring this profound potential for future surgical phases, pushing the boundaries of intelligent assistance (136–138).

- **Enhanced Safety and Automation:** AI harbors the immense potential to fundamentally improve patient safety by continuously monitoring surgical actions, intelligently detecting deviations from planned trajectories, proactively identifying potential hazards, or even predicting complications before they fully manifest in future scenarios. Future applications, such as sophisticated motion analysis, advanced training module enhancement, and intelligent tissue retraction, are being actively explored to dramatically enhance safety and efficiency during complex procedures. Furthermore, AI is set to contribute to increasing levels of robotic autonomy, progressing from supervised control, where the surgeon maintains primary command, to increasingly semi-autonomous tasks where the robot performs specific, pre-programmed maneuvers under human oversight, thereby potentially reducing cognitive load and surgical burden in the future operating room (137,138).

- **Deep Learning for Future Image Recognition and Segmentation:** Deep learning, a powerful subset of AI, is particularly adept and increasingly powerful for advanced image recognition and highly precise semantic segmentation of intricate anatomical structures from complex medical images. This capability enables the creation of highly accurate preoperative 3D models of the liver, allowing for unparalleled precise delineation of tumors, complex vascular structures, and functional liver parenchyma. These sophisticated AI-driven models will be crucial for future patient-specific surgical planning, intelligently guiding resections to achieve clear margins while meticulously preserving maximal functional liver volume (138,140).

Image-Guided Surgery (IGS) in Future Hepatic Robotics: Image-guided surgery itself is undergoing rapid advancements, with future intraoperative imaging technologies, sophisticated navigation systems, and advanced 3D modeling and printing gaining significant prominence for future surgical applications. For robotic liver surgery, IGS is rapidly advancing, with several key modalities showing immense promise in providing profoundly enhanced anatomical and pathological insight in real-time during future complex procedures (141).

- **Advanced 3D Modeling and Navigation Systems:** Future preoperative 3D modeling of the liver, meticulously based on high-resolution CT or MRI scans, will allow surgeons to visualize complex anatomy, including tumor location, intricate vascular structures, and the branching biliary tree, in precise relation to planned resection margins. These meticulously crafted models will then be seamlessly integrated into future intraoperative navigation systems, which will precisely track the position of robotic instruments and dynamically overlay virtual anatomical data directly onto the surgeon's view, intelligently guiding the robotic instruments with sub-millimeter precision through the hepatic parenchyma. The application of advanced 3D visualization technology is crucial for enhancing surgical accuracy in pediatric liver tumors for future interventions, allowing for precise preoperative planning and intraoperative guidance, a principle directly transferable to adult complex cases due to shared anatomical demands (140,141).

- **Integrated Intraoperative Ultrasound (IOUS):** The application of intraoperative ultrasound-guided robotic surgical procedures (RIOUS) is an emerging and highly valuable modality envisioned for future widespread use. RIOUS will leverage the superior ergonomics, enhanced dexterity, and inherent precision of robotic instrumentation to facilitate even more stable and precise manipulation of the ultrasound probe within the abdominal cavity. This improved control will allow for superior real-time tumor localization, precise assessment of resection margins, and highly detailed visualization of deep vascular and biliary structures for future procedures, particularly crucial for lesions not visible on the surface. RIOUS can potentially reduce minimally invasive procedure times and provide thorough assessment at every stage without the need for contrast media or ionizing radiation. This capability is gaining relevance for future general surgery fields, including liver, pancreas, spleen, gallbladder/bile duct, vascular, and rectal surgery, for locating tumors and defining resection margins. It directly addresses and overcomes the limitations of restricted angulation and access inherent in conventional laparoscopic IOUS (97).

- **Advanced Fluorescence Imaging (e.g., Indocyanine Green - ICG):** While ICG fluorescence imaging has found current widespread application, its continued evolution and integration with AI for predictive analysis and profoundly enhanced real-time guidance are definitive future frontiers. Such future fluorescence-guided technologies, including sophisticated near-infrared fluorescence (NIRF), will continue to prove invaluable for various applications in future surgery, helping to identify critical structures, assess tissue viability, and minimize complications (25,83,142).

- **Novel Emerging Optical Imaging Modalities:** The synergistic application of image-guided surgery and robotics is actively leading to the development of highly promising new intraoperative imaging technologies such as optical coherence tomography and confocal laser endomicroscopy. These groundbreaking advancements will allow surgeons to "see through" parenchyma and into vascular structures with unprecedented detail, intelligently avoiding unnecessary dissection by providing a thorough assessment at every stage without the need for contrast media or ionizing radiation (97,141).

The combined and synergistic strength of AI and IGS promises to profoundly revolutionize surgical decision-making and execution in future robotic liver surgery. By consistently providing surgeons with intelligent assistance, advanced predictive insights, and unprecedented real-time anatomical context, these technologies are meticulously setting the stage for even more precise, inherently safer, and ultimately, far more effective hepatic interventions. The overarching future of robotic surgery continues its unwavering aim for the seamless integration and ubiquitous use of advanced image-guided surgery and artificial intelligence. The concept of the future operating room as an intelligent and communicative space platform is gaining significant traction, where fully integrated operating theaters will utilize comprehensive computer platforms to seamlessly merge building data with patient-related data for dramatically enhanced surgical perception and action. This profound integration of vast data and advanced computing is unequivocally expected to further enhance future surgical decision-making and execution, thereby creating a truly adaptive, intelligent, and transformative surgical environment for the ultimate benefit of liver surgery patients (143).

10.2 Augmented Reality, Virtual Reality, and Advanced Robotics

The future trajectory of robotic liver surgery is not solely shaped by artificial intelligence and enhanced image guidance but is also profoundly influenced by the rapidly evolving fields of augmented reality (AR), virtual reality (VR), and the continuous innovation leading to truly advanced, next-generation robotic platforms. These transformative technologies are poised to fundamentally enhance the surgeon's perception, dexterity, and control in future interventions, ultimately pushing the very boundaries of what is achievable in minimally invasive hepatic procedures.

Augmented Reality (AR) in Future Robotic Liver Surgery: Augmented reality involves the dynamic process of overlaying computer-generated virtual images onto a real-world view, thereby profoundly enhancing the surgeon's perception and understanding of the operative field. In the context of future robotic liver surgery, AR promises to deliver a groundbreaking form of "X-ray vision," enabling surgeons to visualize critical anatomical structures and pathological findings that would otherwise remain hidden from direct, visible view (97,141).

- **Enhanced Intraoperative Navigation:** Future AR systems will possess the capability to project sophisticated, real-time three-dimensional (3D) models derived from detailed preoperative imaging (CT, MRI) directly onto the live surgical field as seen through the robotic console. This advanced capability will empower surgeons to "see through" liver parenchyma, allowing for precise identification of tumor margins, visualization of the intricate, often tortuous courses of vital vascular structures (hepatic arteries, portal veins, hepatic veins), and clear delineation of bile ducts that are deeply embedded or obscured. This will fundamentally aid in intelligently avoiding unnecessary dissection, thereby significantly reducing potential blood loss and minimizing iatrogenic injury to vital structures (97,141).

- **Precise Tumor Localization and Resection Planning:** Future AR applications will be instrumental in assisting highly accurate tumor localization, even for minute or deeply seated lesions, by precisely projecting the tumor's exact boundaries onto the liver surface. This will not only facilitate more precise and oncologically sound resections but will also ensure adequate tumor-free margins while meticulously maximizing the preservation of healthy liver tissue, a critical goal in hepatic surgery (88).
- **Guidance for Complex Procedures:** For future complex anatomical resections, such as challenging segmentectomies or those involving centrally located tumors, AR will provide crucial and dynamic guidance for establishing safe dissection planes and understanding complex spatial relationships in real-time. The ongoing application of image-guided surgery and robotics is actively leading to the development of increasingly promising new intraoperative

imaging technologies such as augmented reality itself (88,141).

- **Mitigating Haptic Feedback Limitations:** While current robotic systems may continue to face limitations in providing true haptic feedback, future AR implementations are poised to partially compensate for this by providing highly advanced visual cues and immersive depth information that will significantly enhance spatial perception, thereby potentially reducing the reliance on tactile sensation for precise future tissue discrimination.

Virtual Reality (VR) in Future Robotic Liver Surgery: Virtual reality offers a uniquely immersive experience, completely detaching the user from the physical world and immersing them in a simulated environment. While AR enhances the live surgical field, VR's primary and expanding utility in the future of robotic liver surgery lies in advanced preoperative planning, highly realistic surgical rehearsal, and comprehensive, immersive training programs (50,135).

- **Advanced Surgical Planning and Rehearsal:** Future VR platforms will enable surgeons to conduct exceptionally realistic "dry runs" or rehearsals of complex liver resections, utilizing precise, patient-specific 3D anatomical models. This will empower them to proactively anticipate potential challenges, meticulously plan optimal surgical approaches, and repeatedly rehearse critical maneuvers within a completely risk-free virtual setting, leading to dramatically improved future operative efficiency and a significant reduction in potential intraoperative complications.
- **Enhanced Training and Skill Acquisition:** Future VR simulators will become even more integral components of modern robotic surgery curricula, providing highly controlled and infinitely repeatable environments for advanced skill acquisition. These sophisticated tools will enable trainees to practice highly specific procedural steps and even manage complex simulated complications, thereby accelerating their learning curve and fostering proficiency

without any risk to patients.

- **Patient Education:** Future VR applications can be powerfully utilized to educate patients about their specific liver condition and the proposed robotic surgical procedure, allowing them to visualize their own unique anatomy and the planned intervention with unprecedented clarity and understanding. This will profoundly enhance future patient understanding and facilitate truly informed shared decision-making.

Advanced Robotics Concepts and Future Platforms: Beyond the current iterations of robotic systems, the future of robotic hepatic expansion is characterized by truly emerging designs, innovative functionalities, and expanding capabilities that are predominantly in the research, conceptual, or very early clinical trial phase.

- **Next-Generation Multi-Port Robotic Systems (Future Iterations):** While current multi-port systems are well-established, the future will witness the advent of even more advanced and novel multi-port robotic surgical systems, driving intensified competition and an even more robust push towards further innovation within the robotic surgery landscape (18). These future systems are envisioned with highly modular designs for increased flexibility, open or semi-open consoles for profoundly improved communication within the surgical team, even smaller instruments for broader anatomical access, and a relentless focus on decreased cost, directly addressing persistent financial barriers to widespread adoption (77). The Senhance Surgical System, for instance, with its infrared eye tracking and integrated haptic feedback, represents a current advancement that serves as a foundational step for future iterations(84). The Hugo™ RAS system, with its open console and modular design, offers current advantages that will undoubtedly influence future system designs, such as improved communication and ergonomics, along with enhanced flexibility for multi-quadrant surgeries (89).

- **Future Single-Port Robotic Systems:** The continuous development of single-port robotic systems represents a significant evolutionary trend that will mature further, consistently pushing the boundaries of minimally invasive surgery. Future iterations of platforms like the da Vinci single-port (SP) platform are envisioned to aim for even greater versatility and universal accessibility through a single, smaller incision (90). While current single-port systems offer notable benefits in improved cosmesis and reduced postoperative pain, future developments will further refine these advantages and expand their indications. The SHURUI single-port robotic system stands as a contemporary example of innovation that clearly points towards future directions and enhanced capabilities in single-port robotic surgery (93).
- **Soft Robotics and Micro-Robotics (Conceptual/Early Research):** The distant future may increasingly see the transformative integration of soft robotics, which utilizes

highly compliant materials to navigate exceptionally complex anatomical pathways with unprecedented flexibility and significantly reduced tissue trauma. Furthermore, microscopic robots (micro-robots) and even nanorobots are envisioned for highly localized and targeted interventions, such as ultra-precise drug delivery within the liver parenchyma or microscopic tumor ablation at a cellular level, truly representing uncharted territory in surgical intervention (5).

- **Advanced Haptic Feedback (Robust Implementation):** While some current robotic systems offer limited forms of haptic feedback, a significant and eagerly anticipated future advancement will be the robust and widespread implementation of highly intuitive and genuinely responsive haptic (tactile) feedback in robotic systems. This crucial capability will allow surgeons to feel subtle tissue resistance, accurately differentiate between healthy and diseased tissue, and apply precisely appropriate force during delicate dissection and suturing, thereby profoundly enhancing both safety and precision (31,84).

- **Enhanced Ergonomics (Continued Refinement):** Future robotic systems will continue to prioritize and rigorously refine surgeon comfort and actively reduce physical strain during increasingly prolonged and intricate complex procedures. Newer designs will offer even more advanced adjustable consoles and intuitively designed interfaces, further mitigating the physical demands often associated with traditional surgery (4,10).
- **Synergy and Integrated Operating Rooms of the Future:** The true and transformative power of these future innovations will reside in their profound and dynamic synergy. Advanced AR and VR systems will seamlessly feed rich data into sophisticated AI algorithms for even more intelligent surgical planning and real-time intraoperative guidance, while next-generation robotic platforms will become the exquisitely sophisticated instruments executing

these complex plans with unprecedented precision. The visionary concept of the future operating room as an intelligent and communicative space platform is rapidly gaining significant traction, where fully integrated operating theaters will utilize comprehensive computer platforms to seamlessly merge vast building data with intricate patient-related data for dramatically enhanced surgical perception and optimized action. This profound integration of massive datasets and advanced computing is unequivocally expected to further elevate future surgical decision-making and execution, thereby creating a truly adaptive, intelligently responsive, and ultimately transformative surgical environment for the ultimate benefit of liver surgery patients.

10.3 Role of Robotics in Liver Transplantation and Regenerative Medicine

The transformative potential of robotic surgery, an innovation increasingly driven by precision and advanced visualization, extends beyond standard liver surgery into highly specialized and evolving fields such as liver transplantation and regenerative medicine. These domains present unique complexities where the precise and minimally invasive nature of robotic platforms offers significant promise for improving patient and donor outcomes and advancing scientific frontiers.

While full robotic recipient liver transplantation remains a field of active exploration due to its extreme complexity and the critical need for rapid vascular clamping, robotic assistance is being explored for specific steps. The adoption of minimally invasive techniques in organ transplantation, including the transition from laparoscopic to robotic methods, signifies a notable advancement. Robotic surgery has emerged as a significant development, providing superior precision and outcomes when compared with traditional approaches in these contexts. The inherent advantages of robotic systems, including enhanced dexterity through wristed instruments, superior three-dimensional (3D) visualization, and tremor filtration, provide a level of control and precision that could be highly beneficial for the intricate maneuvers required during recipient hepatectomy and graft implantation. Robotic living donor hepatectomy, in particular, has seen initial exploration, leveraging these advantages.

The intersection of robotics with regenerative medicine opens new avenues for addressing liver disease beyond traditional transplantation. Regenerative medicine aims to repair, replace, or regenerate damaged tissues and organs, often relying on cellular therapies, tissue engineering, and biofabrication. Robotics can provide the extreme precision and controlled movements necessary for highly delicate tasks in tissue engineering, such as automating the seeding of cells onto biodegradable scaffolds or the precise placement of biomaterials to construct functional liver tissue ex vivo. This level of automation ensures reproducibility and scalability in generating complex biological constructs. The precision offered by combining medical science, robotics, and engineering is truly revolutionizing surgical specialties. The integration of robotics into liver transplantation and regenerative medicine is still in its nascent stages but holds immense promise as a future direction for treating hepatic diseases.

10.4 Emerging Platforms and Future Challenges

The trajectory of robotic liver surgery, while already impressive, continues to be shaped by the emergence of new robotic platforms and a persistent landscape of technical, economic, and integration challenges. These dynamics will dictate the pace and direction of future innovations, aiming to further democratize and optimize robotic interventions in hepatic pathologies.

Emerging Robotic Platforms: The singular dominance of the da Vinci Surgical System, which has demonstrated surgical feasibility across numerous procedures since its market introduction in 2000, is increasingly being challenged by a rapidly diversifying market. This proliferation signifies an important evolutionary phase in minimally invasive surgery, characterized by increasing competition and a robust drive towards further innovation within the robotic surgery landscape. Numerous novel multi-port robotic surgical systems are being introduced into clinical practice. Examples of these newer platforms include Micro Hand S, Senhance, Revo-i MSR-5000, KangDuo, Versius, and Hugo™ RAS (19). These new robotic systems often feature modular designs, open or semi-open consoles, smaller instruments, and are frequently developed with the aim of decreasing cost, directly addressing some of the financial barriers to widespread adoption. The Senhance Surgical System, for instance, allows for infrared eye tracking and has integrated haptic feedback, and features an adjustable upright seat, contributing to improved ergonomics (84). The Hugo™ RAS system, with its open console and modular design, offers advantages such as improved communication and ergonomics, along with flexibility for multi-quadrant surgeries (89). This diversification reflects a robust and continuously evolving market actively seeking to provide alternative platforms and to consistently push the boundaries of robotic surgical capabilities even further.

A significant evolutionary trend that will continue to mature is the development of single-port robotic systems. The da Vinci single-port (SP) platform, for example, allows the insertion of three robotic instruments and an articulated scope through a single small incision (90). This design aims to overcome the limitations of both single-incision laparoscopic surgery and traditional multi-port robotic surgery. While currently adopted in various practices, single-port robotic systems offer benefits in terms of improved cosmesis, better postoperative pain control, and decreased length of hospital stay (91,92). These advantages are also being explored and applied in HPB contexts, with robotic biliary surgery utilizing both multiport and single-port cholecystectomy techniques (71). The SHURUI single-port robotic system is another example demonstrating early clinical efficacy and safety in various urologic operations. These systems represent a critical development in minimally invasive surgery, offering potential benefits in cost and pain control compared to traditional multi-port approaches (91).

Future Challenges: Despite the remarkable advancements and the promising trajectory of robotic liver surgery, several key challenges must be addressed to ensure its optimal and equitable global adoption.

- **Cost-Effectiveness:** The inherent high cost associated with the use of the robotic system remains a significant financial barrier that notably limits its widespread adoption. This is primarily driven by the substantial purchase price, ongoing maintenance expenses, and the high cost of disposable instruments. While potential benefits such as more rapid patient recovery and a shorter hospital stay for robotic hepatectomy can partially offset this financial burden, a thorough cost-benefit analysis is continuously necessary. This financial burden is generally expected to decrease in the near future as an increasing number of new surgical systems enter the market, fostering greater competition.
- **Technological Limitations and Refinements:** One notable limitation of early robotic systems was the complete absence of haptic (tactile) feedback, posing considerable technical hurdles for executing highly intricate maneuvers, especially

in delicate and highly vascular environments like the hepatic milieu. While efforts are ongoing to integrate haptic capabilities, its widespread, effective implementation remains a technical challenge. The robotic platform initially remained limited by a paucity of dedicated parenchymal transection devices. The robotic approach often required added operating time associated with docking and instrument exchange.

- **Integration and Interoperability:** As various advanced technologies—AI, AR, IGS, and different robotic platforms—converge, the challenge of seamless integration and interoperability becomes critical. The concept of the future operating room as an intelligent and communicative space platform, where integrated operating theaters utilize comprehensive computer platforms, requires significant advancements in software and hardware integration.
- **Ethical and Regulatory Considerations:** As AI-driven autonomy in robotic surgery increases, new ethical questions

regarding decision-making authority, accountability for errors, and the surgeon's evolving role will arise. Regulatory bodies will need to adapt their frameworks to ensure the safety, efficacy, and ethical deployment of increasingly intelligent and autonomous surgical systems.

- **Evidence Base and Standardization:** Despite promising results and increasing utilization, the evidence base for robotic liver surgery still requires further maturation. There is an ongoing need for large, multicenter, randomized, and prospective studies to definitively analyze the true value and long-term impact of robotic surgery. Standardization of techniques and reporting remains crucial for generating high-quality, comparable data and robust evidence.

The relentless pursuit of innovation, coupled with a concerted effort to address these challenges, will define the future trajectory of robotic liver surgery, promising even greater precision healing and an expanded operative spectrum for patients worldwide.

Conclusion: The Evolving Landscape and Enduring Promise

The narrative meticulously unfolded throughout "The Robotic Revolution in Hepatic Surgery: From Pioneering Scopes to Precision Healing" stands as a profound testament to the transformative power of relentless innovation and the enduring human quest for precision in medicine. What began as audacious conceptualizations of telemanipulation and rudimentary master-slave systems in the latter half of the 20th century, conceived for the austere demands of hazardous or remote environments, has culminated in a profound paradigm shift within the operating theater. This initial genesis, marked by pivotal technological advancements such as the provision of high-resolution three-dimensional (3D) visualization, the ingenious articulation of "endo-wrist" instruments mimicking human dexterity, and the essential filtration of physiological tremor, systematically addressed the inherent limitations of conventional minimally invasive surgery. This technological leap not only enhanced surgical precision but also fundamentally paved the way for robotics to extend its transformative reach into the intricate landscape of Hepato-Pancreato-Biliary (HPB) surgery.

The initial forays of robotics into general abdominal surgery, following crucial regulatory approvals, established critical precedents for feasibility and safety across diverse procedures. These early experiences, while encountering challenges related to the steep learning curve, technical limitations of nascent systems, and the imperative of economic viability, provided invaluable lessons. They illuminated the path for the deliberate and stepwise emergence of robotic liver surgery, a methodical progression distinct from the rapid adoption seen in simpler laparoscopic procedures. This controlled approach allowed for the meticulous identification and resolution of challenges inherent to hepatic intervention, laying the indispensable groundwork for its specialized application.

The subsequent expansion of the operative spectrum in robotic liver surgery has been nothing short of remarkable. What was once confined to minor resections now routinely encompasses major hepatectomies and the intricate management of centrally located and hilar tumors, areas previously considered prohibitive for minimally invasive approaches. The advanced visualization afforded by robotics allows for unparalleled clarity in navigating complex vascular structures and the delicate biliary confluence, optimizing surgical strategy and minimizing complications. Beyond these anatomical complexities, robotic liver surgery has demonstrated its profound utility in treating malignancies. For primary liver cancers (e.g., HCC, cholangiocarcinoma) and colorectal liver metastases, robotic approaches enable meticulous lymphadenectomy and the achievement of critical R0 (negative) resection margins, offering oncological outcomes comparable to traditional open and laparoscopic techniques. This rigorous oncological clearance is further facilitated in challenging contexts, extending the benefits of minimally invasive surgery to previously underserved patient populations. The versatility of the robotic platform has further extended its reach into genuinely challenging and niche scenarios, including the nuanced resection of benign liver tumors, the complex realm of living donor hepatectomy and liver transplantation, acute cases such as liver trauma and other abdominal emergencies, and highly specialized operations in pediatric patients or those presenting with difficult and altered anatomy.

In assessing the current status, robotic liver surgery consistently demonstrates favorable outcomes in terms of reduced blood loss and shorter hospital stays compared to open surgery, with comparable morbidity and mortality rates. The relentless pursuit of standardization in techniques and reporting, guided by international consensus guidelines, remains paramount to ensure patient safety and to build a robust evidence base. Underlying this progress is a critical emphasis on training, education, and simulation. Structured curricula, sophisticated simulation platforms, and comprehensive mentorship programs are indispensable for managing the learning curve and ensuring ongoing surgeon proficiency and competency maintenance in this rapidly evolving field.

Looking towards the horizon, the future of robotic liver surgery is an exhilarating and uncharted territory, poised for profound transformation. The convergence of Artificial Intelligence (AI) and advanced Image-Guided Surgery (IGS) promises to revolutionize surgical decision-making and execution, offering intelligent assistance, predictive insights, and unprecedented real-time anatomical context. The integration of Augmented Reality (AR) and Virtual Reality (VR) will further enhance perception, facilitate highly realistic surgical rehearsal, and refine comprehensive training programs. Concurrently, the continuous evolution of robotic platforms themselves – including next-generation multi-port systems with modular designs, the maturation of single-port robotic systems, the emergence of soft robotics and micro-robotics, and the robust implementation of advanced haptic feedback – will dramatically expand the boundaries of surgical capability. The role of robotics in liver transplantation (both donor and recipient) and regenerative medicine is set for significant expansion, leveraging robotic precision for intricate anastomoses and the manipulation of complex biological constructs.

Despite this exhilarating trajectory, future challenges persist. The high cost of robotic systems, inherent technological limitations (such as the need for universal haptic feedback or specialized instrumentation), and the complexities of seamless integration and interoperability within intelligent operating rooms remain critical hurdles. Ethical and regulatory frameworks must continue to adapt to the increasing autonomy of surgical robots, ensuring patient safety and accountability. Furthermore, a robust evidence base, driven by large, multicenter, randomized controlled trials and rigorous standardization, is indispensable to definitively establishing the true value and long-term impact of robotic surgery across all indications.

In conclusion, "The Robotic Revolution in Hepatic Surgery: From Pioneering Scopes to Precision Healing" is more than a historical account; it is a profound testament to the power of human ingenuity and collaborative scientific endeavor. It underscores how the synergistic efforts of engineers, basic scientists, and surgeons have fundamentally transformed liver surgery from its pioneering scopes to precision healing, consistently offering enhanced safety and tangible patient benefits. The journey is far from complete, but the robust foundation has been firmly laid, setting the stage for an even more adaptive, intelligently responsive, and ultimately transformative surgical landscape that promises a future of enhanced patient care and enduring progress in this vital specialty.

Glossary of Terms

- **3D Vision (Three-Dimensional Vision):** A visualization technology used in robotic surgical systems that provides surgeons with depth perception, mimicking natural human vision and enhancing spatial understanding of the operative field.
- **Anhepatic Phase:** The period during liver transplantation when the diseased liver has been removed and the new liver has not yet been fully revascularized, leading to a temporary absence of liver function.
- **Anastomosis:** A surgical connection made between two tubular structures, such as blood vessels (vascular anastomosis) or bile ducts (biliary anastomosis), crucial in procedures like liver transplantation or gastrointestinal reconstruction.
- **Anatomic Liver Resection:** A surgical technique where a liver segment or section is resected along its vascular and

biliary boundaries, based on precise anatomical principles, often involving Glissonean pedicle isolation.

- **Augmented Reality (AR):** A technology that overlays computer-generated images or virtual information onto a real-world view, enhancing a surgeon's perception of the operative field by providing "X-ray vision" to see hidden structures.
- **Automated Performance Metrics (APMs):** Objective, quantitative measures of surgical technical skills and instrument movements, often derived from robotic system data and used to assess and improve surgeon performance and training.
- **Benign Liver Tumors (BLT):** Non-cancerous growths in the liver, such as hemangiomas, hepatic adenomas, or focal nodular hyperplasia (FNH), that may require surgical removal due to size, symptoms, or diagnostic uncertainty.
- **Biofabrication:** The use of additive manufacturing (3D printing) and other advanced techniques to create biological

tissues, organs, or constructs from cells and biomaterials, often with robotic precision.

- **Biliary Confluence:** The point where multiple bile ducts merge to form larger ducts, crucial anatomical landmarks in liver and HPB surgery, requiring meticulous management to prevent bile leaks.
- **Caudate Lobe:** A deeply situated segment of the liver (Segment I) that has complex vascular relationships, making its surgical resection particularly challenging.
- **Cholangiocarcinoma (CCA):** A primary liver cancer that originates in the bile ducts, often requiring extensive liver resection and lymphadenectomy for oncological clearance.
- **Choledochal Cyst:** A rare congenital dilatation of the bile ducts, a niche pediatric HPB condition that may require surgical excision and reconstruction.
- **Circumferential Resection Margin (CRM):** The radial margin in a resected specimen, especially relevant in rectal cancer surgery, indicating the shortest distance between the

tumor and the cut edge of the tissue; a positive CRM implies residual disease.

- **Clavien-Dindo Classification:** A standardized grading system used to classify the severity of postoperative complications following surgical procedures.
- **Colorectal Liver Metastases (CRLM):** Cancer that has spread from the colon or rectum to the liver, representing a common indication for complex liver resections with curative intent.
- **Competency Maintenance:** The ongoing process by which surgeons sustain and update their skills and knowledge after initial training and credentialing, crucial in a rapidly evolving field like robotic surgery.
- **Conversion to Open Surgery:** The intraoperative decision to switch from a minimally invasive surgical approach (laparoscopic or robotic) to traditional open surgery, typically due to unforeseen complications, anatomical difficulties, or technical challenges.

- **Credentialing:** The formal process by which hospitals or professional bodies grant a surgeon permission to perform specific procedures, based on demonstrated qualifications, training, and competence.
- **da Vinci Surgical System:** A widely adopted robotic surgical platform (e.g., da Vinci Xi, da Vinci SP) known for its master-slave architecture, 3D visualization, and articulated "endo-wrist" instruments, designed to enhance minimally invasive surgery.
- **Dexterity:** The skill and precision in performing movements, particularly with the hands or instruments. Robotic systems enhance dexterity through articulated instruments and motion scaling.
- **Disease-Free Survival (DFS):** A common oncological outcome metric representing the length of time after primary treatment for a cancer that a patient survives without any signs or symptoms of that cancer returning.

- **Docking:** The process of physically connecting the robotic surgical system's arms to the patient's surgical ports, a necessary setup phase for robotic procedures.
- **Economies of Scale:** The concept that increasing the volume of procedures (e.g., in high-volume robotic centers) can lead to a reduction in the average cost per procedure, making expensive technologies more cost-effective.
- **Emerging Platforms:** Newer robotic surgical systems entering or being developed for clinical practice, often featuring modular designs, open consoles, and aiming for reduced costs compared to dominant existing systems.
- **Endo-wrists:** Articulated instruments designed for robotic surgical systems that mimic the natural seven degrees of freedom of the human wrist, providing enhanced maneuverability and precision in confined spaces.
- **Enhanced Recovery After Surgery (ERAS):** Multimodal, evidence-based perioperative care pathways designed to

optimize patient recovery, reduce complications, and shorten hospital stays.

- **Ergonomics:** The science of designing and arranging workplaces and products so that people and things interact most efficiently and safely; in surgery, it relates to surgeon comfort, posture, and reduction of physical strain and fatigue.
- **Feasibility:** The practical possibility of successfully performing a surgical procedure, often demonstrated in early studies of new techniques.
- **Fluorescence Imaging (ICG):** An advanced intraoperative imaging modality, often using Indocyanine Green (ICG) dye, that provides real-time enhanced visualization of vascularity, perfusion, or biliary anatomy, aiding in precise dissection and margin assessment.
- **Focal Nodular Hyperplasia (FNH):** A benign liver tumor, typically asymptomatic, but sometimes requiring resection due to size, symptoms, or diagnostic uncertainty.

- **Glissonean Pedicle Isolation:** A surgical technique for anatomical liver resection involving the isolation and control of Glisson's pedicle (containing branches of the portal vein, hepatic artery, and bile duct) to a specific liver segment.
- **Haptic Feedback:** Tactile or force feedback provided to a surgeon through surgical instruments or console controls, allowing them to "feel" tissue resistance, texture, and tension during a procedure. Many early robotic systems lacked this.
- **Hazardous Environments:** Dangerous settings (e.g., nuclear facilities, battlefields, space) where direct human presence is impractical or unsafe, historically driving the development of telemanipulation.
- **Hemangioma:** The most common type of benign liver tumor, consisting of a tangle of blood vessels. Large hemangiomas may be resected due to size or risk of hemorrhage.

- **Hemostasis:** The process of stopping bleeding during surgery, a critical challenge in highly vascular organs like the liver, where robotic precision is advantageous.
- **Hepatocellular Carcinoma (HCC):** The most common type of primary liver cancer, often arising in the context of chronic liver disease (e.g., cirrhosis), for which surgical resection is a key treatment.
- **Hilar Cholangiocarcinoma (HC):** A type of cholangiocarcinoma located at the hilum of the liver, involving the bile ducts where they exit the liver, presenting significant surgical complexity.
- **Image-Guided Surgery (IGS):** The use of advanced imaging technologies (e.g., 3D models, intraoperative ultrasound, fluorescence imaging) to provide real-time anatomical and pathological information, guiding surgeons during procedures.
- **Indocyanine Green (ICG):** A fluorescent dye used intravenously in fluorescence imaging to visualize vascular

structures, perfusion, and biliary anatomy in real-time during surgery.

- **Intraoperative Ultrasound (IOUS):** The use of ultrasound during surgery to provide real-time imaging of internal structures, aiding in tumor localization, margin assessment, and identification of vessels and ducts.
- **Learning Curve:** The period of time or number of cases required for a surgeon or surgical team to gain proficiency and achieve consistent optimal outcomes with a new surgical technique or technology.
- **Liver Transplantation:** A surgical procedure to replace a diseased or damaged liver with a healthy liver (from a deceased or living donor). Robotic approaches are emerging for donor hepatectomy and recipient procedures.
- **Living Donor Hepatectomy (LDH):** A surgical procedure to remove a portion of the liver from a living donor for transplantation into a recipient. Donor safety is paramount.

- **Lymphadenectomy:** The surgical removal of lymph nodes, typically performed as part of cancer surgery to stage the disease and remove potential metastatic nodes. In HPB surgery, this includes hilar and peripancreatic nodes.
- **Minimally Invasive Surgery (MIS):** Surgical techniques that allow surgeons to perform operations through small incisions, reducing patient trauma, pain, and recovery time compared to traditional open surgery.
- **Motion Scaling:** A feature of robotic systems that translates a surgeon's larger hand movements at the console into smaller, more precise movements of the robotic instruments within the patient, enhancing fine motor control.
- **Multi-Degree-of-Freedom (Multi-DOF):** Refers to instruments (like robotic endo-wrists) that can move and articulate in multiple planes, mimicking the flexibility of the human hand and wrist.
- **Niche Scenarios:** Specific, often less common, or highly complex patient populations or clinical situations that

present unique challenges for surgical intervention (e.g., pediatric patients, liver trauma, patients with difficult anatomy).

- **Oncological Clearance (R0 Resection):** The primary goal in cancer surgery, meaning that the entire tumor has been removed with clear (negative) margins, indicating no cancer cells are left behind at the edge of the resected tissue.
- **Overall Survival (OS):** An oncological outcome metric representing the length of time from diagnosis or start of treatment that patients with cancer are still alive.
- **Parenchymal Transection:** The process of cutting through the liver tissue during a hepatectomy, a highly critical step due to the liver's vascularity and fragility.
- **Pediatric Surgery:** A surgical subspecialty focusing on the surgical care of infants, children, and adolescents, often involving smaller anatomical spaces and delicate tissues, presenting unique challenges for robotic application.

- **Pneumoperitoneum:** The inflation of the abdominal cavity with gas (typically carbon dioxide) during laparoscopic and robotic surgery to create a working space for instruments and visualization.
- **Posterior-Superior Segments:** Anatomically challenging segments of the liver (Segments VII and VIII) are located high and posteriorly, notoriously difficult to access and resect with conventional minimally invasive approaches.
- **Prognosis:** The likely course of a medical condition or disease, often assessed in cancer patients using various factors, including surgical outcomes.
- **R0 Resection:** See Oncological Clearance.
- **Regenerative Medicine:** A field of medicine focused on repairing, replacing, or regenerating damaged tissues and organs, often involving cellular therapies, tissue engineering, and biofabrication, where robotics can play a role in precision.

- **Remote Presence:** The sensation or ability of a human operator to feel as if they are physically present at a distant location while controlling a robotic system.
- **Robotic-Assisted Surgery (RAS):** Surgical procedures performed with the aid of a robotic system, where the surgeon controls instruments from a console, benefiting from enhanced visualization and dexterity.
- **Robotic Hepatectomy (RH):** The surgical removal of part of the liver using a robotic surgical system.
- **Senhance Surgical System:** An alternative multi-port robotic surgical platform known for features like eye-tracking camera control and integrated haptic feedback.
- **Single-Port Robotic Systems (SP):** Robotic surgical platforms that allow all instruments and the camera to be inserted through a single, small incision, aiming for improved cosmesis and reduced pain.

- **Telemanipulation:** The control of a machine or robot from a distance, a foundational concept for surgical robotics initially explored for hazardous environments.
- **Tremor Filtration:** A feature of robotic surgical systems that filters out and eliminates the natural physiological tremors of a surgeon's hands, resulting in more stable and precise instrument movements.
- **Virtual Reality (VR):** A technology that immerses a user in a completely simulated environment, often used in surgical training and preoperative planning for realistic rehearsal.
- **ZEUS Robotic Surgical System:** An early robotic surgical system that received FDA approval, contributing to the initial landscape of surgical robotics before the widespread dominance of the da Vinci system.

References

1. Szijártó A, Lévay K, Pekli D. [The path leading to robotic surgery]. Magy Onkol. 2024 Sep 19;68(3):201–5.

2. Lane T. A short history of robotic surgery. Ann R Coll Surg Engl. 2018 May;100(6_sup):5–7.

3. Dohrn N, de Heer P, Burgdorf SK, Jensen KK, Klein MF, Gögenur I. [The application, rationale, and current evidence for a robotic approach in abdominal surgery]. Ugeskr Laeg. 2022 Sep 5;184(36).

4. Minamimura K, Hara K, Matsumoto S, Yasuda T, Arai H, Kakinuma D, et al. Current status of robotic gastrointestinal surgery. J Nippon Med Sch. 2023;90(4):308–15.

5. Püschel A, Schafmayer C, Groß J. Robot-assisted techniques in vascular and endovascular surgery. Langenbeck's Arch Surg. 2022 Aug;407(5):1789–95.

6. Hazey JW, Melvin WS. Robot-assisted general surgery. Semin Laparosc Surg. 2004 Jun;11(2):107–12.

7. Hatcher AJ, Beneville BT, Awad MM. The evolution of surgical skills simulation education: Robotic skills. Surgery. 2025 May;181:109173.

8. Spiegelberg J, Iken T, Diener MK, Fichtner-Feigl S. Robotic-Assisted Surgery for Primary Hepatobiliary Tumors-Possibilities and Limitations. Cancers (Basel). 2022 Jan 6;14(2).

9. Salloum C, Lim C, Malek A, Compagnon P, Azoulay D. Robot-assisted laparoscopic liver resection: A review. J Visc Surg. 2016 Dec;153(6):447–56.

10. Materazzi G, Rossi L. Robot-assisted adrenalectomy: state of the art. Updates Surg. 2021 Jun;73(3):1131–46.

11. El-Hakim A, Tewari A. Robotic prostatectomy - a review. MedGenMed. 2004 Oct 25;6(4):20.

12. Higuchi N, Kanno K, Onji H, Masuda S, Taniguchi R, Ochi Y, et al. Comparing approaches to benign hysterectomy using conventional multi-port and newer single-port robots: a propensity score matching analysis of surgical outcomes and literature review. J Robot Surg. 2025 Jun 23;19(1):320.

13. Lenfant L, Canlorbe G, Belghiti J, Kreaden US, Hebert AE, Nikpayam M, et al. Robotic-assisted benign hysterectomy compared with laparoscopic, vaginal, and open surgery: a systematic review and meta-analysis. J Robot Surg. 2023 Dec;17(6):2647–62.

14. Solaini L, Cavaliere D, Avanzolini A, Rocco G, Ercolani G. Robotic versus laparoscopic inguinal hernia repair: an updated systematic review and meta-analysis. J Robot Surg. 2022 Aug;16(4):775–81.

15. Crestani A, Merlot B, Denost Q, Francois MO, Assenat V, Lacheray IC, et al. [Colorectal endometriosis surgery: Technical and technological innovations in service of a complex surgery]. Gynecol Obstet Fertil Senol. 2025 Jun;53(6):298–305.

16. Mikhail E, Pavlovic ZJ, Al Jumaily M, Kheil MH, Moawad GN, Soares T. Robot-Assisted Surgery for Endometriosis: Current and Future Perspectives. Surg Technol Int. 2022 May 19;40:197–202.

17. Xu M-Y, Song Z-Y, Liang C-Z. Robot-assisted repair of ureteral stricture. J Robot Surg. 2024 Sep 28;18(1):354.

18. Cowan B, Gomes C, Morris P, Fryrear R, Petraiuolo W, Walton M, et al. Robotic technology in surgery: a classification system of soft tissue surgical robotic devices. Surg Endosc. 2024 Jul;38(7):3645–53.

19. Leang YJ, Kong JCH, Mosharaf Z, Hensman CS, Burton PR, Brown WA. Emerging multi-port soft tissue robotic systems: a systematic review of clinical outcomes. J Robot Surg. 2024 Mar 30;18(1):145.

20. Robinson TN, Stiegmann GV. Minimally invasive surgery. Endoscopy. 2004 Jan;36(1):48–51.

21. Idrees K, Bartlett DL. Robotic liver surgery. Surg Clin North Am. 2010 Aug;90(4):761–74.

22. Fahrner R, Rauchfuß F, Bauschke A, Kissler H, Settmacher U, Zanow J. Robotic hepatic surgery in malignancy: review of the current literature. J Robot Surg. 2019 Aug;13(4):533–8.

23. Tu Y, Jiang J, Huang J, Sui J, Yang S. A review of wrist mechanism design and the application in gastrointestinal minimally invasive surgery of multi-degree-of-freedom surgical laparoscopic instruments. Surg Endosc. 2025 Jan;39(1):99–121.

24. Arezzo A, Vettoretto N, Francis NK, Bonino MA, Curtis NJ, Amparore D, et al. The use of 3D laparoscopic imaging systems in surgery: EAES consensus development conference 2018. Surg Endosc. 2019 Oct;33(10):3251–74.

25. Gonzalez-Ciccarelli LF, Quadri P, Daskalaki D, Milone L, Gangemi A, Giulianotti PC. Robotic approach to hepatobiliary surgery. Chirurg. 2017 Jan;88(Suppl 1):19–28.

26. Minamimura K, Aoki Y, Kaneya Y, Matsumoto S, Arai H,

Kakinuma D, et al. Current status of robotic hepatobiliary and pancreatic surgery. J Nippon Med Sch. 2024 Mar 9;91(1):10–9.

27. Shimizu A, Ito M, Lefor AK. Laparoscopic and Robot-Assisted Hepatic Surgery: An Historical Review. J Clin Med. 2022 Jun 7;11(12).

28. Myla K, Bou-Ayash N, Kim WC, Bugaev N, Bawazeer M. Is implementation of robotic-assisted procedures in acute care general surgery cost-effective? J Robot Surg. 2024 May 27;18(1):223.

29. Guerra F, Di Marino M, Coratti A. Robotic surgery of the liver and biliary tract. J Laparoendosc Adv Surg Tech A. 2019 Feb;29(2):141–6.

30. Muaddi H, Hafid ME, Choi WJ, Lillie E, de Mestral C, Nathens A, et al. Clinical outcomes of robotic surgery compared to conventional surgical approaches (laparoscopic or open): A systematic overview of reviews. Ann Surg. 2021 Mar 1;273(3):467–73.

31. Ayabe RI, Azimuddin A, Tran Cao HS. Robot-assisted liver resection: the real benefit so far. Langenbecks Arch Surg. 2022 Aug;407(5):1779–87.

32. Lafaro KJ, Stewart C, Fong A, Fong Y. Robotic Liver Resection. Surg Clin North Am. 2020 Apr;100(2):265–81.

33. Caba Molina D, Lambreton F, Arrangoiz Majul R. Trends in robotic pancreaticoduodenectomy and distal pancreatectomy. J Laparoendosc Adv Surg Tech A. 2019 Feb;29(2):147–51.

34. Straatman J, Pucher PH, Knight BC, Carter NC, Glaysher MA, Mercer SJ, et al. Systematic review: robot-assisted

versus conventional laparoscopic multiport cholecystectomy. J Robot Surg. 2023 Oct;17(5):1967–77.

35. Klimeczek-Chrapusta M, Stolarz K, Preinl M, Bogusz B, Gruba M, Górecki W. Robot-assisted vs. laparoscopic Nissen fundoplication in children: an updated meta-analysis with systematic literature review. J Robot Surg. 2025 May 6;19(1):202.

36. Hegazy M, Toubasey S, Giudice FD, Challacombe B. Contemporary Practice in Adrenal Surgery: A Review of Multiport versus Single-port and Transperitoneal versus Retroperitoneal Approaches. Eur Urol Focus. 2025 Jan;11(1):26–8.

37. Arang H, El Boghdady M. Robotic Appendicectomy: A review of feasibility. Sultan Qaboos Univ Med J. 2023 Nov 30;23(4):440–6.

38. Saqib SU, Bajwa AA. The role of Da Vinci Xi robotic simulation curriculum in enhancing skills in robotic colorectal surgery. Ann Med Surg (Lond). 2023 Dec;85(12):6001–7.

39. Pathak A, Wanjari M. Minimally invasive colorectal surgery techniques. Cureus. 2023 Oct 17;15(10):e47203.

40. Liao B, Xue X, Zeng H, Ye W, Xie T, Wang X, et al. Comparison of different surgical techniques and anastomosis methods in short-term outcomes of right colon cancer: a network meta-analysis of open surgery, laparoscopic, and robot-assisted techniques with extracorporeal and intracorporeal anastomosis. Updates Surg. 2025 Apr;77(2):309–25.

41. Marano L, Cwalinski T, Girnyi S, Skokowski J, Goyal A, Malerba S, et al. Evaluating the role of robotic surgery

gastric cancer treatment: A comprehensive review by the Robotic Global Surgical Society (TROGSS) and european federation international society for digestive surgery (EFISDS) joint working group. Curr Oncol. 2025 Jan 31;32(2).

42. Guerrini GP, Esposito G, Magistri P, Serra V, Guidetti C, Olivieri T, et al. Robotic versus laparoscopic gastrectomy for gastric cancer: The largest meta-analysis. Int J Surg. 2020 Oct;82:210–28.

43. Izumi D, Nunobe S. How to decide approaches and procedures for early and advanced gastric cancer? Can J Gastroenterol Hepatol. 2022 Apr 4;2022:8324242.

44. Ilic D, Evans SM, Allan CA, Jung JH, Murphy D, Frydenberg M. Laparoscopic and robotic-assisted versus open radical prostatectomy for the treatment of localised prostate cancer. Cochrane Database Syst Rev. 2017 Sep 12;9(9):CD009625.

45. Stockheim J, Perrakis A, Sabel BA, Waschipky R, Croner RS. RoCS: Robotic Curriculum for young Surgeons. J Robot Surg. 2023 Apr;17(2):495–507.

46. Wong SW, Crowe P. Factors affecting the learning curve in robotic colorectal surgery. J Robot Surg. 2022 Dec;16(6):1249–56.

47. Vining CC, Skowron KB, Hogg ME. Robotic gastrointestinal surgery: learning curve, educational programs and outcomes. Updates Surg. 2021 Jun;73(3):799–814.

48. Vierstraete M, Simons M, Borch K, de Beaux A, East B, Reinpold W, et al. Description of the current da vinci® training pathway for robotic abdominal wall surgery by the

European Hernia Society. J Abdom Wall Surg. 2022 Nov 30;1:10914.

49. Flynn J, Larach JT, Kong JCH, Waters PS, Warrier SK, Heriot A. The learning curve in robotic colorectal surgery compared with laparoscopic colorectal surgery: a systematic review. Colorectal Dis. 2021 Nov;23(11):2806–20.

50. Rahimi AO, Ho K, Chang M, Gasper D, Ashouri Y, Dearmon-Moore D, et al. A systematic review of robotic surgery curricula using a contemporary educational framework. Surg Endosc. 2023 Apr;37(4):2833–41.

51. Larkins K, Khan M, Mohan H, Warrier S, Heriot A. A systematic review of video-based educational interventions in robotic surgical training. J Robot Surg. 2023 Aug;17(4):1329–39.

52. Awad L, Reed B, Bollen E, Langridge BJ, Jasionowska S, Nikkhah D, et al. Does robotic surgery have a role in abdominal wall reconstruction? A systematic review and meta-analysis. J Plast Reconstr Aesthet Surg. 2025 Jul;106:353–92.

53. Poulsen JL, Bruun B, Oestergaard D, Spanager L. Factors affecting workflow in robot-assisted surgery: a scoping review. Surg Endosc. 2022 Dec;36(12):8713–25.

54. Liu R, Abu Hilal M, Wakabayashi G, Han H-S, Palanivelu C, Boggi U, et al. International experts' consensus guidelines on robotic liver resection in 2023. World J Gastroenterol. 2023 Aug 28;29(32):4815–30.

55. Flemming S, Wiegering A, Germer CT, Reibetanz J. [Robotic adrenalectomy-current evidence]. Chirurgie (Heidelb). 2024 Oct;95(10):810–7.

56. Keller DS, Jenkins CN. Safety with Innovation in Colon and Rectal Robotic Surgery. Clin Colon Rectal Surg. 2021 Sep 3;34(5):273–9.

57. Rosen SA, Rupji M, Liu Y, Paul Olson TJ. Robotic proctectomy: beyond the initial learning curve. Am Surg. 2023 Dec;89(12):5332–9.

58. Khan AU, Khan A, Danial A. Robotic versus laparoscopic approaches to distal pancreatectomy: quality assessment of the current evidence. J Coll Physicians Surg Pak. 2025 May;35(5):628–35.

59. Anyomih TTK, Mehta A, Sackey D, Woo CA, Gyabaah EY, Jabulo M, et al. Robotic versus laparoscopic general surgery in the emergency setting: a systematic review. J Robot Surg. 2024 Jul 5;18(1):281.

60. De Nagy J, Youssef Y, Moawad G. Strategies and factors to maximize cost-effectiveness of robotic surgery in benign gynecological disease. Best Pract Res Clin Obstet Gynaecol. 2023 Aug;90:102380.

61. Bai F, Li M, Han J, Qin Y, Yao L, Yan W, et al. More work is needed on cost-utility analyses of robotic-assisted surgery. J Evid Based Med. 2022 Jun 18;15(2):77–96.

62. Williamson T, Song S-E. Robotic surgery techniques to improve traditional laparoscopy. JSLS. 2022;26(2).

63. Fernandes E, Giulianotti PC. Robotic-assisted pancreatic surgery. J Hepatobiliary Pancreat Sci. 2013 Aug;20(6):583–9.

64. Boggi U, Caniglia F, Amorese G. Laparoscopic robot-assisted major hepatectomy. J Hepatobiliary Pancreat Sci. 2014 Jan;21(1):3–10.

65. Sugioka A, Kato Y, Tanahashi Y. Systematic extrahepatic Glissonean pedicle isolation for anatomical liver resection based on Laennec's capsule: proposal of a novel comprehensive surgical anatomy of the liver. J Hepatobiliary Pancreat Sci. 2017 Jan;24(1):17–23.

66. Di Benedetto F, Petrowsky H, Magistri P, Halazun KJ. Robotic liver resection: Hurdles and beyond. Int J Surg. 2020 Oct;82S:155–62.

67. Tsekouras K, Spartalis E, Mamakos N, Tsourouflis G, Nikiteas NI, Dimitroulis D. The use of robotics in surgery of benign liver diseases: A systematic review. Surg Innov. 2022 Apr;29(2):258–68.

68. Del Angel Millan G, Cassese G, Giannone F, Del Basso C, Alagia M, Lodin M, et al. Postoperative outcomes after robotic liver resection of caudate lobe: A systematic review. Medicina (Kaunas). 2024 Dec 29;61(1).

69. Giannone F, Cassese G, Del Basso C, Alagia M, Palucci M, Sangiuolo F, et al. Robotic versus laparoscopic liver resection for difficult posterosuperior segments: a systematic review with a meta-analysis of propensity-score matched studies. Surg Endosc. 2025 Jan;39(1):64–76.

70. Delgado LM, Pompeu BF, Pasqualotto E, Magalhães CM, Oliveira AFM, Kato BK, et al. Robotic-assisted cholecystectomy versus conventional laparoscopic cholecystectomy for benign gallbladder disease: a systematic review and meta-analysis. J Robot Surg. 2024 Jun 5;18(1):242.

71. Chang K, Gokcal F, Kudsi OY. Robotic Biliary Surgery. Surg Clin North Am. 2020 Apr;100(2):283–302.

72. Alfonso A, McFarland KN, Savsani K, Lee S, Imai D, Khan

A, et al. Robotic management of primary cholecystoduodenal fistula: A case report and brief literature review. Int J Med Robot. 2024 Apr;20(2):e2629.

73. Magistri P, Tarantino G, Assirati G, Olivieri T, Catellani B, Guerrini GP, et al. Robotic liver resection for hepatocellular carcinoma: A systematic review. Int J Med Robot. 2019 Aug;15(4):e2004.

74. Vancoillie S, Willems E, De Meyere C, Parmentier I, Verslype C, D'Hondt M. Robotic versus laparoscopic repeat hepatectomy: A comparative single-center study of perioperative outcomes. Eur J Surg Oncol. 2025 Jan;51(1):109376.

75. Liu Q, Li M, Gao Y, Jiang T, Han B, Zhao G, et al. Effect of robotic versus open pancreaticoduodenectomy on postoperative length of hospital stay and complications for pancreatic head or periampullary tumours: a multicentre, open-label randomised controlled trial. Lancet Gastroenterol Hepatol. 2024 May;9(5):428–37.

76. Hobeika C, Pfister M, Geller D, Tsung A, Chan AC-Y, Troisi RI, et al. Recommendations on Robotic Hepato-Pancreato-Biliary Surgery. The Paris Jury-Based Consensus Conference. Ann Surg. 2025 Jan 1;281(1):136–53.

77. Choi SB, Choi SY. Current status and future perspective of laparoscopic surgery in hepatobiliary disease. Kaohsiung J Med Sci. 2016 Jun 1;32(6):281–91.

78. Choi JH, Diab A-R, Tsay K, Kuruvilla D, Ganam S, Saad A, et al. The evidence behind robot-assisted abdominopelvic surgery: a meta-analysis of randomized controlled trials. Surg Endosc. 2024 May;38(5):2371–82.

79. Guerrini GP, Lauretta A, Belluco C, Olivieri M, Forlin M,

Basso S, et al. Robotic versus laparoscopic distal pancreatectomy: an up-to-date meta-analysis. BMC Surg. 2017 Nov 9;17(1):105.

80. Harrell KN, Kooby DA. Laparoscopic pancreatic resection. Minerva Chir. 2015 Oct;70(5):355–64.

81. Neshan M, Padmanaban V, Chick RC, Pawlik TM. Open vs robotic-assisted pancreaticoduodenectomy, cost-effectiveness and long-term oncologic outcomes: a systematic review and meta-analysis. J Gastrointest Surg. 2024 Nov;28(11):1933–42.

82. Poppinga J, Ritter AS, Steinkraus KC, Nießen A, Hackert T. Surgery of Early-Stage Pancreatic Cancer. Visc Med. 2025 May 15;1–7.

83. Wang X, Teh CSC, Ishizawa T, Aoki T, Cavallucci D, Lee S-Y, et al. Consensus guidelines for the use of fluorescence imaging in hepatobiliary surgery. Ann Surg. 2021 Jul 1;274(1):97–106.

84. McKechnie T, Khamar J, Daniel R, Lee Y, Park L, Doumouras AG, et al. The senhance surgical system in colorectal surgery: A systematic review. J Robot Surg. 2023 Apr;17(2):325–34.

85. Campetella M, Ragonese M, Gandi C, Bizzarri FP, Russo P, Foschi N, et al. Surgeons' fatigue in minimally invasive and open surgery: A review of the current literature. Urologia. 2025 Feb;92(1):161–8.

86. Wee IJY, Kuo L-J, Ngu JC-Y. A systematic review of the true benefit of robotic surgery: Ergonomics. Int J Med Robot. 2020 Aug;16(4):e2113.

87. Tetteh E, Wang T, Kim JY, Smith T, Norasi H, Van Straaten

MG, et al. Optimizing ergonomics during open, laparoscopic, and robotic-assisted surgery: A review of surgical ergonomics literature and development of educational illustrations. Am J Surg. 2024 Sep;235:115551.

88. Baldari L, Boni L, Cassinotti E. Hybrid robotic systems. Surgery. 2024 Nov;176(5):1538–41.

89. Romero-Marcos JM, Sánchez-Romero A, González-Abós S, Cuenca-Gómez C, Sánchez-Guillén L, Sampson-Dávila JG, et al. Application of the Hugo™ RAS robotic system in general surgery: a scoping review. J Robot Surg. 2025 Jun 14;19(1):289.

90. Celotto F, Ramacciotti N, Mangano A, Danieli G, Pinto F, Lopez P, et al. Da Vinci single-port robotic system: current application and future perspective in general surgery: A scoping review. Surg Endosc. 2024 Sep;38(9):4814–30.

91. Nguyen TT, Basilius J, Ali SN, Dobbs RW, Lee DI. Single-Port Robotic Applications in Urology. J Endourol. 2023 Jun;37(6):688–99.

92. Hasan O, Reed A, Shahait M, Crivellaro S, Dobbs RW. Robotic surgery for stone disease. Curr Urol Rep. 2023 Mar;24(3):127–33.

93. Li Z-Y, Luo C. Perioperative outcomes of the SHURUI single-port robotic system in urologic surgery: a systematic review and single-arm meta-analysis. J Robot Surg. 2025 Jun 30;19(1):334.

94. Lengyel BC, Chinnadurai P, Corr SJ, Lumsden AB, Bavare CS. Robot-assisted vascular surgery: literature review, clinical applications, and future perspectives. J Robot Surg. 2024 Aug 23;18(1):328.

95. Rompianesi G, Montalti R, Giglio MC, Caruso E, Ceresa CD, Troisi RI. Robotic central pancreatectomy: a systematic review and meta-analysis. HPB (Oxford). 2022 Feb;24(2):143–51.

96. Stefanova I, Vescio F, Nickel F, Merali N, Ammendola M, Lahiri RP, et al. What are the true benefits of robotic pancreaticoduodenectomy for patients with pancreatic cancer? Expert Rev Gastroenterol Hepatol. 2024 May 10;18(4–5):133–9.

97. Pavone M, Seeliger B, Teodorico E, Goglia M, Taliento C, Bizzarri N, et al. Ultrasound-guided robotic surgical procedures: a systematic review. Surg Endosc. 2024 May;38(5):2359–70.

98. Becher E, Jericevic D, Huang WC. Minimally Invasive Surgery for Patients with Locally Advanced and/or Metastatic Renal Cell Carcinoma. Urol Clin North Am. 2020 Aug;47(3):389–97.

99. Tamhane N, Roberts B, Wiegand L, Mikhail E. Robotic surgery for urologic deep infiltrating endometriosis: A review and case presentations. Surg Technol Int. 2020 Nov 28;37:154–60.

100. Broering DC, Raptis DA, Malago M, Clavien P-A, MIOT Collaborative. Revolutionizing organ transplantation with robotic surgery. Ann Surg. 2024 Nov 1;280(5):706–12.

101. Dutta S, Khan AS, Ukeje CC, Chapman WC, Doyle MB, Scherer M, et al. Anesthetic considerations for robotic liver transplantation. J Cardiothorac Vasc Anesth. 2025 Jun;39(6):1571–82.

102. Finotti M, D'Amico F, Testa G. The current and future role of robotic surgery in liver surgery and transplantation.

Minerva Surg. 2022 Aug;77(4):380–90.

103. Dincer HA, Dogrul AB. Advances in minimally invasive liver surgery. North Clin Istanb. 2024 Nov 20;11(6):586–92.

104. Di Sandro S, Centonze L, Ratti F, Russolillo N, Conci S, Gringeri E, et al. Robotic vs laparoscopic resection for hepatocellular carcinoma: multicentric propensity-score matched analysis of surgical and oncologic outcomes in 647 patients. Updates Surg. 2025 Jul 20;

105. Cillo U, D'Amico FE, Furlanetto A, Perin L, Gringeri E. Robotic hepatectomy and biliary reconstruction for perihilar cholangiocarcinoma: a pioneer western case series. Updates Surg. 2021 Jun;73(3):999–1006.

106. Wang W, Fei Y, Liu J, Yu T, Tang J, Wei F. Laparoscopic surgery and robotic surgery for hilar cholangiocarcinoma: an updated systematic review. ANZ J Surg. 2021 Jan;91(1–2):42–8.

107. Dong S, Jiang A, An S, Xiao J. Comparison of robot-assisted, open, and laparoscopic-assisted surgery for cholangiocarcinoma: a network meta-analysis. Langenbecks Arch Surg. 2024 Nov 8;409(1):336.

108. Chee MYM, Wu AGR, Fong K-Y, Yew A, Koh YX, Goh BKP. Robotic, laparoscopic and open surgery for gallbladder cancer: a systematic review and network meta-analysis. Surg Endosc. 2024 Sep;38(9):4846–57.

109. Wang J, Li Z, Chen L-L, Zhao J-B, Wu J-L, Leng Z-W. Comparing robotic and open surgical techniques in gallbladder cancer management: a detailed systematic review and meta-analysis. J Robot Surg. 2024 Mar 5;18(1):111.

110. Liu F, Wu Z-R, Hu H-J, Jin Y-W, Ma W-J, Wang J-K, et al. Current status and future perspectives of minimally invasive surgery in gallbladder carcinoma. ANZ J Surg. 2021 Mar;91(3):264–8.

111. Rocca A, Scacchi A, Cappuccio M, Avella P, Bugiantella W, De Rosa M, et al. Robotic surgery for colorectal liver metastases resection: A systematic review. Int J Med Robot. 2021 Dec;17(6):e2330.

112. Chang W, Ye Q, Xu D, Liu Y, Zhou S, Ren L, et al. Robotic versus open surgery for simultaneous resection of rectal cancer and liver metastases: a randomized controlled trial. Int J Surg. 2023 Nov 1;109(11):3346–53.

113. Baek S-J, Piozzi GN, Kim S-H. Optimizing outcomes of colorectal cancer surgery with robotic platforms. Surg Oncol. 2021 Jun;37:101559.

114. Khan MH, Tahir A, Hussain A, Monis A, Zahid S, Fatima M. Outcomes of robotic versus laparoscopic-assisted surgery in patients with rectal cancer: a systematic review and meta-analysis. Langenbecks Arch Surg. 2024 Sep 3;409(1):269.

115. Ishizuka M, Shibuya N, Hachiya H, Nishi Y, Kono T, Takayanagi M, et al. Robotic surgery is associated with a decreased risk of circumferential resection margin positivity compared with conventional laparoscopic surgery in patients with rectal cancer undergoing mesorectal excision: A systematic review and meta-analysis. Eur J Surg Oncol. 2024 Oct;50(10):108538.

116. Takamoto T, Mihara Y, Nishioka Y, Ichida A, Kawaguchi Y, Akamatsu N, et al. Surgical treatment for hepatocellular carcinoma in the era of multidisciplinary strategies. Int J Clin Oncol. 2025 Mar;30(3):417–26.

117. Kossenas K, Kouzeiha R, Moutzouri O, Georgopoulos F. Comparing the operative, oncological, post-operative outcomes and complications of robotic and laparoscopic pancreaticoduodenectomy for the treatment of pancreatic and periampullary cancers: a systematic review and meta-analysis with subgroup analysis. J Robot Surg. 2025 Mar 5;19(1):97.

118. Zhang W, Huang Z, Zhang J, Che X. Safety and efficacy of robot-assisted versus open pancreaticoduodenectomy: a meta-analysis of multiple worldwide centers. Updates Surg. 2021 Jun;73(3):893–907.

119. Leitao MM, Kreaden US, Laudone V, Park BJ, Pappou EP, Davis JW, et al. The RECOURSE Study: Long-term Oncologic Outcomes Associated With Robotically Assisted Minimally Invasive Procedures for Endometrial, Cervical, Colorectal, Lung, or Prostate Cancer: A Systematic Review and Meta-analysis. Ann Surg. 2023 Mar 1;277(3):387–96.

120. Horgan S, Vanuno D, Sileri P, Cicalese L, Benedetti E. Robotic-assisted laparoscopic donor nephrectomy for kidney transplantation. Transplantation. 2002 May 15;73(9):1474–9.

121. Broering DC, Elsheikh Y, Alnemary Y, Mahmood A, Majeed A, Marcos A, et al. Improved Short-Term Outcomes With Fully Robotic Recipient Adult Living Donor Liver Transplantation: A Comparative Study. Ann Surg. 2025 Jun 20;

122. Ceccarelli G, Catena F, Avella P, Tian BW, Rondelli F, Guerra G, et al. Emergency robotic surgery: the experience of a single center and review of the literature. World J Emerg Surg. 2024 Aug 17;19(1):28.

123. Wu J, Martin MJ, Kirkpatrick V, Cassaro S, Pérez Rodríguez

F. The great debate: robotic vs traditional surgical approach in the acute care setting. Am Surg. 2024 Oct;90(10):2357–61.

124. Rusch R, Hoffmann G, Rusch M, Cremer J, Berndt R. Robotic-assisted abdominal aortic surgery: evidence and techniques. J Robot Surg. 2022 Dec;16(6):1265–71.

125. Esposito C, Cerulo M, Lepore B, Coppola V, D'Auria D, Esposito G, et al. Robotic-assisted pyeloplasty in children: a systematic review of the literature. J Robot Surg. 2023 Aug;17(4):1239–46.

126. Gundeti MS, Huberman-Shlaes J. Robotics in pediatric urology: A review. J Pediatr Surg. 2025 Mar;60(3):162022.

127. Zhang M-X, Chi S-Q, Cao G-Q, Tang J-F, Tang S-T. Comparison of efficacy and safety of robotic surgery and laparoscopic surgery for choledochal cyst in children: a systematic review and proportional meta-analysis. Surg Endosc. 2023 Jan;37(1):31–47.

128. Zhang R, Liu S, Li T, Zhan J. Efficacy of robot-assisted hepaticojejunostomy and laparoscopic-assisted hepaticojejunostomy in pediatric congenital choledochal dilatation: a system review and meta-analysis. Pediatr Surg Int. 2022 Dec 11;39(1):46.

129. Jacobson JC, Scrushy MG, Gillory LA, Pandya SR. Utilization of robotics in pediatric surgical oncology. Semin Pediatr Surg. 2023 Feb;32(1):151263.

130. Ferrero PA, Blanc T, Binet A, Arnaud A, Abbo O, Vatta F, et al. The potential and the limitations of esophageal robotic surgery in children. Eur J Pediatr Surg. 2022 Apr;32(2):170–6.

131. Chen Y-C, Tsai Y-Y, Ke T-W, Shen M-Y, Fingerhut A, Chen WT-L. Robotic versus laparoscopic pelvic lateral lymph node dissection in locally advanced rectal cancer: a systemic review and meta-analysis. Surg Endosc. 2024 Jul;38(7):3520–30.

132. Hannan E, Feeney G, Ullah MF, Amin K, Coffey JC, Peirce C. The first robotic transanal minimally invasive surgery in Ireland: a case-based review. Ir J Med Sci. 2022 Apr;191(2):853–7.

133. Wang J, Johnson NW, Casey L, Carne PWG, Bell S, Chin M, et al. Robotic colon surgery in obese patients: a systematic review and meta-analysis. ANZ J Surg. 2023 Jan;93(1–2):35–41.

134. Yang L-W, Bai X-Y, Jing G-M. Systematic review and meta-analysis of short-term outcomes: robot-assisted versus laparoscopic surgery for gastric cancer patients with visceral obesity. J Robot Surg. 2024 Jun 4;18(1):238.

135. Bramhe S, Pathak SS. Robotic surgery: A narrative review. Cureus. 2022 Sep 15;14(9):e29179.

136. Boal MWE, Anastasiou D, Tesfai F, Ghamrawi W, Mazomenos E, Curtis N, et al. Evaluation of objective tools and artificial intelligence in robotic surgery technical skills assessment: a systematic review. Br J Surg. 2024 Jan 3;111(1).

137. Moglia A, Georgiou K, Georgiou E, Satava RM, Cuschieri A. A systematic review on artificial intelligence in robot-assisted surgery. Int J Surg. 2021 Nov;95:106151.

138. Urbanski A, Babic B, Schröder W, Schiffmann L, Müller DT, Bruns CJ, et al. [New techniques and training methods for robot-assisted surgery and cost-benefit analysis of Ivor

Lewis esophagectomy]. Chirurg. 2021 Feb;92(2):97–101.

139. Han J, Davids J, Ashrafian H, Darzi A, Elson DS, Sodergren M. A systematic review of robotic surgery: From supervised paradigms to fully autonomous robotic approaches. Int J Med Robot. 2022 Apr;18(2):e2358.

140. Dong Q, Xiu W, Tang B, Hiyama E, Austin MT, Wu Y, et al. International multidisciplinary consensus recommendations on clinical application of three-dimensional visualization in precision surgery for pediatric liver tumors. HPB (Oxford). 2025 Jun;27(6):733–45.

141. Makary J, van Diepen DC, Arianayagam R, McClintock G, Fallot J, Leslie S, et al. The evolution of image guidance in robotic-assisted laparoscopic prostatectomy (RALP): a glimpse into the future. J Robot Surg. 2022 Aug;16(4):765–74.

142. Patel NM, Patel PH, Yeung KTD, Monk D, Mohammadi B, Mughal M, et al. Is robotic surgery the future for resectable esophageal cancer?: A systematic literature review of oncological and clinical outcomes. Ann Surg Oncol. 2024 Jul;31(7):4281–97.

143. Teber D, Engels C, Maier-Hein L, Ayala L, Onogur S, Seitel A, et al. [Surgery 4.0-are we ready?]. Urologe A. 2020 Sep;59(9):1035–43.

Index

A

B

C

K

L

M

N

O

P

R

www.ingramcontent.com/pod-product-compliance
Lightning Source LLC
LaVergne TN
LVHW060027210926
848481LV00013B/3808